D1712280

Development of Electronic Aids for the Visually Impaired

Documenta Ophthalmologica Proceedings Series

Development of Electronic Aids for the Visually Impaired

Proceedings of a workshop on the Rehabilitation of the Visually Impaired, held at the Institute for Research on Electromagnetic Waves of the National Research Council, Florence, Italy. Sponsored by the Commission of the European Communities as advised by the Committee on Medical and Public Health Research

Edited by P.L. Emiliani

Istituto di Ricerca sulle Onde
Ellettromagnetiche del Consiglio
Nazionale delle Ricerche,
Florence, Italy

1986 **MARTINUS NIJHOFF/DR W. JUNK PUBLISHERS**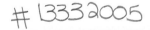
a member of the KLUWER ACADEMIC PUBLISHERS GROUP
DORDRECHT / BOSTON / LANCASTER
for the COMMISSION OF THE EUROPEAN COMMUNITIES

Distributors

for the United States and Canada: Kluwer Academic Publishers, 190 Old Derby Street, Hingham, MA 02043, USA
for the UK and Ireland: Kluwer Academic Publishers, MTP Press Limited, Falcon House, Queen Square, Lancaster LA1 1RN, UK
for all other countries: Kluwer Academic Publishers Group, Distribution Center, P.O. Box 322, 3300 AH Dordrecht, The Netherlands

Library of Congress Cataloging in Publication Data

ISBN 0-89838-805-8 (this volume)
EUR 10103 EN

Book information

Publication arranged by: Commission of the European Communities, Directorate-General Information Market and Innovation, Luxembourg

Copyright/legal notice

PRINTED IN THE NETHERLANDS

FOREWORD

This book is based on the papers presented at the Workshop
on "Rehabilitation of the Visually Impaired" held in Florence at the Institute for the Research on Electromagnetic
Waves of the Italian Research Council on April 4-6, 1984.

The Workshop, sponsored by the Committee for Medical and
Public Health Research of the Commission of the European
Communities, was meant to exchange ideas about the need,
importance and feasibility of a European cooperation in
the field of visual impairment and to identify promising
research areas, where current national activities could
take advantage of such a collaboration in order to increase
their efficiency. In particular, it dealt with the development and use of technical aids (mainly based on computers
and signal processing techniques) and with the elaboration,
evaluation and standardization of new methods and tests.

The attendance was multidisciplinary, including researchers
from the fields of technology, medicine and psychology and
representatives from organizations involved in the rehabilitation of the visually impaired. Five technical sessions
were organized, dealing with the following topics: automatic
production of Braille and systems for paperless Braille,
aids for reading and for the interaction with coded information sources, low vision aids, transduction of visual information into a tactile representation, mobility aids.
Three different application sectors were mainly considered:
education and culture, vocational training, mobility.
A final session was devoted to a discussion in working groups.
The results are briefly outlined in the following concise
report of the Workshop.

Thanks to the wide attendance and to the high level and en-
thusiasm of the participants, the book gives up-to-date
information about the state of the art of the activity and
about the trends in this sector in the European countries.

I should like to express my thanks to all the participants,
who willingly cooperated to set up the Workshop in a very
short time and coordinated their presentations in order to

have a balanced program. In particular, I should like to
express my gratitude to Dr. D.H.A. Aberson (Eindhoven),
Prof. G. Bruun (Lingby), Dr. D.J. Powell (London), Dr. A.
Sargentini Daniele (Roma), Dr. M. Truquet (Toulouse),
members of the Planning Group, who helped in the preparation of the proposal of the Workshop, to Dr. W. Skupinski
of the EEC Commission, who continuously supported the organization, to Dr. G.R. Bock, Project Leader of the Hearing
Impairment Program, who gave us important information about
his program, to Dr. M. Stilmant of the Bureau for Action
of Disabled People, to Prof. V. Cappellini, Director of IROE,
who allowed us to use the facilities of the Institute and
supported the organization of the meeting, to my colleagues
Dr. P. Graziani and Dr. A. Tronconi, who joined in the local
organizing committee, to Dr. I. Campo, who helped in the
setting up of the program, to Mr. A. Gabbanini, Mr. F. Meiners,
Mr. F. Poli, Mr. M. Tesi, Mr. L. Zuccagnoli, from the technical staff of the Institute, who helped in the different phases
of the organization, and to Mrs. V. Cammelli who made really
possible to set up the Workshop with her secretarial activity.

                                        Pier Luigi Emiliani

Firenze, April 1985

WELCOME TO THE PARTICIPANTS

I am very glad to open the works of this Workshop of European Communities on "Rehabilitation of Visually Impaired", giving my best welcome to all the Participants from different European Nations.

The program of the Workshop is very intense and interesting, covering the most important areas of Rehabilitation of Visually Impaired with significant contributions in the following areas: Braille production, Aids for reading and for the interaction with coded information sources, Low-Vision, Transduction of visual information and displays for the blind, Mobility.

We are very happy to have this important Workshop at our Institute, which is strongly involved in the field, both at national level in the Finalized Project "Biomedical Technologies", chaired by Prof. L. Donato, and at the European level.

I am sure that your works will give a significant contribution to the covered field in Europe, contributing to obtain an higher level of cooperation and interaction in this research area of Commission of the European Communities.

Thanking Dr. P.L. Emiliani and his cooperators for the very active organization of this Workshop, I wish to all of you the best success for your works and the most enjoying visit to Florence.

Vito Cappellini

CONTENTS

XII

LIST OF PARTICIPANTS

Aberson D.H.A., Institute for Perception Research, P.O. Box 513,
5600 MB Eindhoven, The Netherlands

Bock G.R., EEC Hearing Impairment Programme Project Leader, MRC
Institute of Hearing Research, University of Nottingham, University
Park, Nottingham NG7 2RD, U.K.

Bruel A., ENSEEIHT, 2 rue Camichel, 31071 Toulouse Cedex, France

Bruun G., Electronics Laboratory, Electronics Institute, Technical
University of Denmark, Bldg. 344, DK-2800 Lyngby, Denmark

Campo I.M., Centro "David Chiossone", Corso Armellini, 11,
16122 Genova, Italy

Da Ronch A., LADSEB - C.N.R., Corso Stati Uniti, 4, 35100 Padova, Italy

Doove H., Netherlands Library for the Blind, Zichtenburglaan 260,
2544 EB The Hague, The Netherlands

Dubus J.P., Université des Sciences et Techniques de Lille, Laboratoire
de Mesures Automatiques, Batiment P3, 59655 Villeneuve d'Ascq Cedex, France

Emiliani P.L., Istituto di Ricerca sulle Onde Elettromagnetiche (I.R.O.E.),
C.N.R., Via Panciatichi, 64, 50127 Firenze, Italy

François G., Katholieke Universiteit Leuven, Departement Elektrotechniek,
Kardinaal Mercierlaan 94, B-3030 Leuven Heverlee, Belgium

Gill J.M., Research Unit for the Blind, Brunel University, Uxbridge,
Middlesex UB8 3PH, U.K.

Granström B., Department of Speech Communication and Music Acoustics,
Royal Institute of Technology, S-10044 Stockholm, Sweden

Graziani P., Istituto di Ricerca sulle Onde Elettromagnetiche (I.R.O.E.),
C.N.R., Via Panciatichi,64, 50127 Firenze, Italy

Hache J.C., Coorganizer of a related Workshop on Visual Impairment,
Service d'Esploration Fonctionnelle de la Vision, Hôpital Central de
Lille, 6900 Lille, France

Hamonet C., COMAC-BME Representative, Chef de Service de Rééducation Fonctionnelle, Hôpital Henri Mondor, F-94010 Creteil Cedex, France

Harres M., Deutsche Blindenstudienanstalt, Am Schlag 8, Postfach 11 60, D-3550 Marburg/Lahn, German Federal Republic

Heyes A.D., Blind Mobility Research Unit, University of Nottingham, Nottingham NG7 2RD, U.K.

Jansson G., Department of Psychology, University of Uppsala, P.O. Box 227, S-751 04 Uppsala, Sweden

King R.W., Department of Electronics and Information Engineering, University of Southampton, Highfield, Southampton SO9 5NH, U.K.

Levett J., Athens School of Public Health, 196 Alexandra Ave., Athens 11522, Greece

Lirou P., Université Paul Sabatier, Laboratoire L.S.I., 118, Route de Narbonne, 31062 Toulouse Cedex, France

Mandar A., Université des Sciences et Techniques de Lille, Laboratoire de Mesures Automatiques, Batiment P3, 59655 Villeneuve d'Ascq Cedex, France

Orban G.A., Katholieke Universiteit Leuven, Laboratorium voor Neuro -en Psychofysiologie, Campus Gasthuisberg, Herestraat, B-3000 Leuven, Belgium

Pedotti A., COMAC-BME Representative, Centro di Bioingegneria, Politecnico di Milano, Via Gozzadini, 7, 20148 Milano, Italy

Powell D.J., Moorfields Eye Hospital, City Road, London EC1V 2PD, U.K.

Sargentini Daniele A., COMAC-BME Representative, Direttore Laboratorio Ingegneria Biomedica, Istituto Superiore di Sanità, Viale Regina Elena, 299, 00161 Roma, Italy

Silver J., Moorfields Eye Hospital, City Road, London EC1V 2PD, U.K.

Skupinski W., Commission of the European Communities, Directorate-General for Science, Research and Development, 200 Rue de la Loi, B-1049 Bruxelles, Belgium

Soede M., Institute for Rehabilitation Research, Zandbergsweg 111, 6432 CC Hoensbroek, The Netherlands

Sørensen J.A., Electronics Laboratory, Electronics Institute, Technical University of Denmark, Bldg. 344, DK-2800 Lyngby, Denmark

Stilmant M., Commission of the European Communities, Bureau for Action in Favour of Disabled People, Directorate-General for Employment, Social Affairs and Education, 200 Rue de la Loi, B-1049 Bruxelles, Belgium

Thomsen P., Institute for the Blind, Studiebogsbibliotek for Blinde (Students' Library), Rymarkvej 1, DK-2900 Hellerup, Denmark

Tobin M.J., Research Centre for the Education of the Visually Handicapped, University of Birmingham, 59 Selly Wick Road, Birmingham, B29 7JE, U.K.

Truquet M., Centre TOBIA, Université Paul Sabatier, 118, Route de Narbonne, 31062 Toulouse Cedex, France

Walraven J., Institute for Perception TNO, Kampweg 5, 3769 ZG Soesterberg, The Netherlands

Warburg M., The Copenhagen Eye Clinic for the Mentally Retarded, Gentofte Hospital, 40, Sognevej, DK-2820 Gentofte, Denmark

Werner H., Institut für Angewandte Mathematik, University Bonn, Wegelerstr. 6, D-5300 Bonn, German Federal Republic

OBSERVERS:

Coppens A., Katholieke Universiteit Leuven, B-3000 Leuven, Belgium

Hertlein J., Deutsche Blindenstudienanstalt, Am Schlag 8, D-3550 Marburg, German Federal Republic

Quatraro A., Stamperia Braille, Regione Toscana, Via Fibonacci, 9, 50131 Firenze, Italy

Soldati A., Istituto Ciechi, Via Vivaio, 7, 20122 Milano, Italy

Spinabelli R., LADSEB/CNR, Corso Stati Uniti, 4, 53100 Padova, Italy

Susini C., Istituto di Ricerca sulle Onde Elettromagnetiche (I.R.O.E.), C.N.R., Via Panciatichi, 64, 50127 Firenze, Italy

Swinnen T., Katholieke Universiteit Leuven, B-3000 Leuven, Belgium

Testa A., Centro "David Chiossone", Corso Armellini, 11, 16122 Genova, Italy

Timpano A., Regione Toscana, Via L.C. Farini, 8, 50121 Firenze, Italy

Tronconi A., Istituto di Ricerca sulle Onde Elettromagnetiche (I.R.O.E.), C.N.R., Via Panciatichi, 64, 50127 Firenze, Italy

Ventura E., IPSIA Ciechi "A. Nicolodi", Via V. Emanuele II, 2, 50134 Firenze, Italy

CONCISE REPORT
Workshop on Rehabilitation of the Visually Impaired
Florence, April 4-6, 1984

P.L. Emiliani
Chairman of the Planning Group and of the local organizing committee

The Workshop on "Rehabilitation of the Visually Impaired" was proposed an an exploratory activity to develop ideas about the feasibility of a European collaboration in the field of visual impairment. In particular, it was organized to bring together researchers from the fields of technology, medicine and psychology and representatives from the organizations involved in rehabilitation to discuss about the development and use of technical aids (mainly based on computers and signal processing techniques) and about the elaboration, evaluation and standardization of new rehabilitation methods and tests.

Blind and visually impaired people can benefit from recent technological advances if some problems, related to the use of technology, are correctly recognized and solved, such as, for instance, the following:

a) careful identification of the type and degree of disability;
b) careful evaluation of the needs of the visually disabled;
c) critical evaluation of existing aids and usable technology;
d) development of an efficient training for the use of the different aids;
e) development of suitable rehabilitation programs based on the available aids;
f) coordination between the development and testing of aids and their introduction in actual rehabilitation programs;
g) assessment of methods for matching or prescribing aids to the users in different situations, including the multiple disabled;
h) matching of the rehabilitation approaches and used aids with the expectations of the disabled people.

A coordinated effort for a correct use of technology is now particularly important, since recent developments in electronics and the diffusion of low-cost microcomputers and computerized equipment seem to offer new possibilities in the production of technical aids. The use of standardized devices (microcomputers) and of new emerging technology (e.g. synthetic speech) can lead to a reduction in the cost of these aids and to an increase in their reliability, ease of maintenance and matching to the needs of individual users.

The correct use of technology is connected with a multidisciplinary approach to the rehabilitation process, where the development of aids has to start from the identification of the real needs of the disabled and their use has to be finalized to their integration in the society.

Therefore, a multidisciplinary attendance to the workshop was sought for, so that the problems could be considered from different points of view: technical, medical, psychological, sociological, etc. Moreover, the workshop was organized to consider both the problems of low vision patients and totally blind people, with respect to the following application fields:
- education and culture;
- vocational training;
- mobility.

Three main sectors of interest were identified in the preparatory meetings, namely:
- the communication sector, including all the methodology to transduce visual information into a form suitable for its transfer through a sensory channel as an alternative to the lacking one;
- the low vision sector, where visual aids are normally preferred to substitutive ones;
- the mobility sector.

Due to the complexity and wide range of the different techniques to be considered in the first sector, it was decided to split it in three different sessions:
1) automatic production of Braille and systems for paperless Braille;
2) aids for reading and for the interaction with coded information sources;
3) transduction of visual information into a tactile representation.

Contributions were required not only to present relevant results in rehabilitation, but also to review the state of the art in this sector and to point out problems for further efforts in research and development on a concerted basis.

Therefore, papers were requested to describe results obtained in:
- implementation of technical aids;
- rehabilitation techniques;
- evaluation of technology and rehabilitation techniques;
- research in progress in new technology;
taking into account, when possible and/or applicable, several factors, such as, for example:
- identification of disabilities and demographics;
- training for the use of aids;
- perceptual aspects;
- testing procedures for the evaluation of the rehabilitation level;
- impact of the rehabilitation techniques in education and access to culture;

- relevance in vocational training;
- problems in the production and diffusion of aids.

A last session was devoted to the discussion in working groups to point out the main problems in the different sectors (communication, low vision and mobility) and to prepare proposals for further activity. In a final plenary session the conclusions of the working groups were discussed.

In session 1 the problems of Braille production were considered. The following items were presented and discussed:
- implementation of software for the production of grade 2, scientific and musical Braille;
- production from compositor tapes;
- impact of new technology in the automatic production of Braille (optical character reading, character recognition, voice recognition, etc.);
- devices for Braille production;
- devices for paperless Braille (Braille word processors).

A lot of problems were pointed out for further discussion and development, namely:
- standardization of scientific and musical Braille;
- standardization of the software for Braille formatting and production;
- copyright problems in the use of compositor tapes and need of efficient software interfaces with the different formats of tapes;
- efficent use of new technology (e.g. character recognition versus compositor tapes);
- standardization of the supports and of the interaction software for paperless Braille word processors;
- maintenance problems.

In session 2 the peripheral devices for the communication of the blind with coded information sources (computers, data banks, general information systems, as teletex, etc.) and the related interaction methodology were considered, such as:
- interaction systems based on paperless Braille;
- interaction systems based on synthetic speech;
- speech synthesizers;
- reading machines for the blind.

General technical requirements were pointed out during the discussions, such as the following:
- reduction in cost and complexity and increase in quality of the speech synthesizers for general use;
- increase in reliability and quality of the ephemeral Braille presentation systems and study of new presentation formats (e. g. a Braille page) and technology;
- study of efficient techniques for character reading and recognition, incorporating also results from artificial intelli-

gence;
- standardization of the interaction protocols and interaction software.

Moreover, some general requirements were also emphasized:
- critical evaluation of the interaction protocols and the involved technology;
- field tests, performed by independent persons different from the designers;
- tests on the acceptance of the products and on the adaptation to the human user;
- trade-off between the use of technology and the use of other rehabilitation forms;
- analysis of the impact of technology on social integration (access to culture, vocational training and so on).

As a general observation, the convenience of the use, when possible, of technology and devices available and developed for general use was pointed out.

In session 3 the main problems (clinical, social, psychological and technological) of low vision patients were considered, such as the perceptual aspects of reading, the assessment of the needs of the patients, the necessity of interfaces between research and users of its results, the organization of prescription and diffusion of aids.

Several points were established such as the following:
- the high percentage of the partially sighted compared with the blind in the population of visually handicapped;
- the preference of the partially sighted for visual aids rather than substitutive ones;
- the need of recognizing the diversities in the population of the partially sighted and hence the difference in needs;
- the necessity of an assessment of the influence of magnification (major type of solution for the partially sighted) on the reading gain in acuity (perception of single letters), on the scanning procedure and the field size (more short-time memory required);
- the need of a multidisciplinary approach;
- the necessity of a careful definition of blindness;
- the importance of training for the use of low vision aids.

In session 4 the following items were presented and discussed:
- development of tactile-acoustic and multimodal graphical displays;
- interactive presentation of graphical information;
- impact of image processing techniques on the transduction of images for the blind and the visually impaired;
- development of computer graphics for the blind;
- compatibility and acceptability of the information presented to the human brain;

- development of models of the three main sensory channels (vision, hearing, touch) to improve the design of artificial sensory channels.
    The main problems pointed out were the following:
- need of new technology to develop more efficient graphical displays;
- limited knowledge of the tactile perceptual system;
- relationship among the economical implications in the development of sensory aids and the difficulties in the diffusion of technology among the blind population;
- need of a multidisciplinary approach, involving blind users, in the development of aids;
- opportunity of searching common areas of interest in the development of vision substitution systems and other fields of research as robot vision and artificial intelligence.

    In session 5 the problems connected with the study, implementation and evaluation of aids and methodology for mobility were considered, such as:
- review of the main available mobility aids;
- long cane versus electronic mobility aids;
- new approaches to the development of mobility aids;
- perceptual aspects and general problems of the mobility of the blind.
    The following aspects of mobility were pointed out:
- importance of the long cane;
- unsatisfactory performance of the existing electronic mobility aids;
- insufficient knowledge about the information necessary for mobility and its presentation form;
- psychological versus engineering approach;
- opportunity of the evaluation of both prototypes and already existing mobility aids in an artificial rather than in a natural environment.

    In the last afternoon three working groups were organized to prepare comments and proposals for a future coordinated activity: a communication group (Dr. P.L. Emiliani), a low vision group (Dr. J. Silver) and a mobility group (Dr. A. Heyes). The recommendations of the three working groups are reported in the following pages.

A) Communication aids

Field of interest: devices and methodology for the transduction
of information (coded, written, graphical) to be transferred
through an alternative sensory channel.

1) Proposal to discover the existing usage of communication aids
   within the European countries;
   a) types of used transduction forms (interfaces);
   b) training;
   c) use in education and vocational training.

2) Proposal to stimulate and coordinate research in the following areas:
   a) transduction of written information:
      a1) paper Braille (standardization of the formatting and
          production software, automatic production from compos-
          itor tapes or using optical readers);
      a2) paperless Braille (standardization of the supports,
          interaction software);
      a3) automatic reading machines (input - image acquisition,
          character recognition; output - Braille, synthetic
          speech);
   b) interaction with coded information sources (computers, da-
      ta banks);
   c) transduction of graphical information:
      c1) devices for tactile drawing production;
      c2) perceptual aspects;
      c3) image processing (e.g. image simplification and fea-
          ture extraction);
      c4) impact of computer graphics techniques;
      c5) standardization of symbols and presentation formats;
   d) integration of the different means for the presentation
      of information and methodology for an user-friendly inter-
      facing (hardware and software) with the different aids;
   e) possibilities in education and vocational training, due to
      the impact of technology on society and on the production
      of aids.

3) Proposed workshops:
   - Standardization of interfaces (input-output)
   - Job changing
   - Multihandicaps
   - Application of modern electronic devices in the revision,
     editing and production of textbooks and educational materi-
     al in Braille.

B) Low vision

1) Proposal to establish a model for the development and delivery of low vision services within the countries of the EEC.

2) Proposal to establish a multidisciplinary European group, to have a free exchange of information and research on:
   - epidemiology;
   - technology;
   - methodology;
   - sociology;
   - psychology;
   - education;
   - clinical assessment.

C) Mobility group

1) Proposal to discover the existing usage of aids within the European countries:
   a) types of devices in use;
   b) available training;
   c) institute responsible;
   d) who finances the issue of the aids.

2) Proposal to stimulate and coordinate research in the following areas:
   a) perceptual guidance of walking;
   b) neuro-physiological aspects;
   c) hardware development:
      c1) information gathering;
      c2) information processing;
      c3) information display;
   d) evaluation.

3) Identification of workers in these areas.

4) Dissemination of information about the activity.

5) Exchange of information between the different countries.

6) Proposed workshops:
   Mobility workshop.

Session 1: BRAILLE PRODUCTION

Chairman: M. Truquet

Automatic Production of Braille
M. Truquet

Progress in Automatic Production of Braille
H. Werner

Automatic Production of Braille - A Danish Experience
P. Thomsen

Innovation, Braille Information and Workplace Design
M. Soede

Necessary Priority Areas in the Development of Technical
Aids for the Blind in the Federal Republic of Germany
M. Harres

The Elekul Braille System
G. François

Written Communication Aids Between Sighted and
Non Sighted Persons
J.P. Dubus, A. Mandar, M. Mortreux, F. Wattrelot

Discussion

AUTOMATIC PRODUCTION OF BRAILLE

M. TRUQUET

Centre de Transcription et d'Edition en Braille (TOBIA)
Laboratoire Langages et Systèmes Informatiques,
Université Paul Sabatier, Route de Narbonne, 118 -
31062 TOULOUSE - FRANCE.

INTRODUCTION

Each year we observe that the need for Braille is increasing thanks to the compulsory attendance for the blind, some of whom are even coming to the University to attend courses in higher education. But, for their studies, the blind need Braille (grade 2 or scientific Braille) and in many cases the computer can provide these rapid transcriptions. To be efficient a complete Braille edition system is necessary but as it is very expensive, it is difficult to get.

I - THE AUTOMATIC BRAILLE PRODUCTION

Why use a computer for Braille production? Because the computer allows:

Good Braille to be obtained with only the help of a typist who does not know Braille systems; advantage to be taken of text editor systems, to make the work of the typist easier; the user to be able to choose among different storages; a Braille document to be transcribed rapidly; networks access, and thus access to data banks.

I - 1: The Braille edition:

To obtain very good Braille we have to follow the usual practice of newpapers' editors:

The document entered by the typist or from a compositors' tape must be proofread.

Then corrected.

Then transcribed.

Then the Braille document must be proofread by a blind person (who must have perfect knowledge of Braille systems). At TOBIA Center all Braille documents are proofread before being published, because some difficulties occur when we have to represent a figure on a Braille document and only a blind person can decide how this should be done.

Then we proceed to the Braille print or the large print.

N.B.

(I) As regards the compositors' tapes there is still no standard among printing houses; moreover not all publishers archive their final corrected version (normally they prefer to correct the galley proofs). These considerations give many opportunities for the optical readers, in fact they will use documents without mistakes and those produced by the optical reader are notified by the system on the screen so it is easy to correct them.

(II) Concerning the special codes used to indicate italics, proper names, indented lines, etc... some of them must be introduced by a typist in every case, whether the origin of the document is a data bank, compositor's tape, optical reader, etc...

1.2 Target applications :
In many areas:
- . cultural: novels, poems, cultural news, etc...
- . education: handbooks, university documents, exam subjects etc...
- . general information: newpapers, magazines, trade-union documents, messages, invitations etc...
- . professional life: office notes, job information, etc...
- . daily life: bank statements, medicine information,etc...

N.B.: Handbooks and university documents cannot be transcribed like this. Often some visual information has to be described and added to the text. So manual entering is preferred. As regards novels, the optical reader can be used with no problems if there are no footnotes.

II SOFTWARE FOR BRAILLE FORMATTING
From one year to another microcomputers become cheaper. So it is important to realize portable programs to give the blind the same benefits as the sighted person.

With a computer and several programs it is possible for a Braille editor centre to produce Braille in many areas but also to carry out other tasks. That aim imposes programs written in a language like PASCAL or FORTRAN used by several computers. These are the languages in common use at the present time. But for future programs it will be important that a commission decide what computer language to choose according to the evolution of microcomputers (why not ADA?).

What sort of software?
2.1 Evidently a program to transcribe literature into Braille (grade 1 and grade 2). A program as perfect as possible able to transcribe even groups of words separated by several spaces as in French "POUR AINSI DIRE" (so-to-speak) which is abbreviated PAD. (We must not forget that a word processor, used by the typist, places many spaces to justify the line).

2.2 A program to transcribe mathematics or scientific documents into Braille. We have to define the means used to type the scientific document. For example, in Toulouse we use a HP 2644, a terminal provided with mathematic generator characters and cartridges units. The whole system depends on that device. As the cartridges are not reliable, we have to think of another process to continue our experiment. Certainly we will use an HP device with the same mathematical generator characters which includes 255 mathematic symbols obtained thanks to the three keyboards:

One for subscripts and superscripts,
one for logical, relational and functional operators,
one for the Greek alphabet.

(Only the record on a file of the entered document will be different).

The operator has to reproduce the exact image of the original document on the screen. There is no hierarchy for the writing, the screen being registered on the cartridge or other magnetic record only when it is full.

The first job the program has to do is to try to determine the main line (the text being scanned vertically from top to bottom and from left to right). Then the program divides the expression into several data groups according to the meeting of "-" and "+" as intermediary characters.

The following algorithm represents the general process of linearization:

WHILE   **(not end of text)**

DO BEGIN
    determine next data group;
    determine the main line of this group;

  WHILE   **(not end of line)**

  DO BEGIN
    determine next horizontal group;
    determine this horizontal group;
    concatenate the linearized text
  END

  END

When the scientific expression is linearized the program for Braille transcription is called for. The program proceeds in two steps:

- In the first step only the mathematical expression is considered, linearized then transcribed into Braille. That Braille document will only be read by the second step and formatted by the Braille text editor.

- In the second step the literary text in transcribed into Braille grade 2 to be formatted by the Braille text editor with the scientific Braille document. This system can transcribe a general or a specialized scientific text. For each specialization we only have to change the mathematical table. This system makes possible the use of compositor's tapes.

2.3 A program to transcribe music into Braille: the usual (manual) production of scores is heavy and difficult. The transcriber must be able to read a staff and have a perfect knowledge of the Braille music system. Two years are necessary to acquire a good knowledge of Braille so the Braille production for music is poor.

At TOBIA the system used is an interactive system. The program can detect syntactic and semantic mistakes (incomplete measure, inconceivable octave value, etc...). When an error is detected a message is printed and an arrow indicates the point where the error is found. The operator brings in the modifications and if no mistakes are detected he is then able to reproduce the score on a graphic visual display, and compare it to the original.

Braille music is the same in every country, only the presentation changes. The program is able to give two presentations:
. bar after bar: used by English language speaking countries,
. fragment by fragment: used by French musicians.

As regards the input of a score, the language implemented tries to satisfy the following criteria:
. easier learning,
. easier utilisation,
. easier proofreading and correction
. easier evolution of the language used.

2.4   A program to realize the grade 1 transcription from a grade 2 transcription then print it on to an ink-print display. This program is running on a DIGITAL Equipment Computer, it will be implemented on the BULL DPS8 MULTICS and on the ORDIBRAILLE. It will be used by students to re-read their exam before the output on an ink-print display.

Remarks concerning the TOBIA programs:
1. The Braille literary program is written in FORTRAN IV, it was formerly written in Assembly language. Since 1970 it has been running on IBM computers, CII computers (IRIS 80 for example), and now on a BULL computer, a DPS8 MULTICS. It can be called from a MINITEL through TRANSPAC network. A new version, again in FORTRAN, is being prepared to be used on microcomputers.

2. The Braille mathematical program is written in PASCAL language and it is running on an ALPHA microsystem minicomputer. As the visual display HP2644A has some failures we have stopped the experiment for a while.

3. The transcription from grade 2 to grade 1 program is written in PASCAL language; it is running on a DIGITAL equipment minicomputer. A new version is being prepared to be used on the ORDIBRAILLE.

4. The Braille transcription program of music is written in PASCAL language; it is running on an ALPHA microsystem minicomputer and it will also be adapted to run on a BULL DPS8 MULTICS.

III EQUIPMENT FOR BRAILLE PRODUCTION :
To obtain a Braille document it is necessary to have at least the following devices available:
. a computer or microcomputer
. a visual display
. a ink-print-display
. a Braille printer

As regards the Braille printer we have to distinguish two sorts of production.

3.1 A medium production:

This corresponds to the punctual Braille production. For that, we have at the present time the following devices
- the BRAILLO (2) from Norway:
  . the Braillo 270 which allows 800 pages per hour to be obtained;
  . the Braillo 400 which allows 1200 pages per hour to be obtained.

These devices are capable of obtaining interpoint which allows reduction in volume of the books and at the same time the price of the books. It uses paper of 120gsm (weight).

- the ELEKUL (7) from Belgium (Pr François):
  400 c/s (1200 pages per hour).
  It uses paper of 160gsm, not fanfold paper, but continuous paper.

- the RESUS (RS14) (10)
  It embosses 300 lines per minute.
  It uses fanfold paper of 160gsm (weight).

3.2 A large print :

For these, two devices are necessary:
- an embossing machine like:
  . the PUMA ESV (5) from West Germany. It embosses (metal plates) ten characters per second. It can be directly connected to a computer.
  . the PED 30 (13) from United States. It embosses 30 characters per second and it is directly connected to any computer.

- a press:
  (A special paper placed between both plates is pressed in order to obtain the Braille document). The best known are those of MARBURG (5). We have to mention the rotative press which embosses 7000 signatures per hour.

3.3 As regards the individual devices we should mention, among those used at the present time :

- the SAGEM device (11) French. It embosses 15 characters per second. The interpoint is possible.

- The LED 120 (13) from the United States. it embosses 120 characters per second.

- The BRAILLO 20 (2) from Norway. It embosses 20 characters per second.

- The Cranmer modified PERKINS (8). It embosses 10 characters per second. It does not use fanfold paper and it is possible to obtain graphics and figures.

IV EQUIPMENT FOR PAPERLESS BRAILLE

Many devices are used at the present time or are near to being used. They are very expensive because the manufacturers wish to provide a complete system (able to read, write etc..).

Three years ago ELINFA produced, for the LIBRARY of CONGRESS, a reader only, not so expensive and for a library it is sufficient. Why not follow up that experience and build in at the same time a single device and a special device with many functions able to help the Blind when they will have to consult a data bank or to do anything else?
At the present time we have to mention the following devices:
- the BRAILLEX (9) from West Germany (Papenmeir) with 32 Braille tactile characters: the BRAILLEX C which uses cassettes, the BRAILLEX D which uses floppy disks. Characters, the BRAILLEX System:
It uses many functions:
. the record function: which allows the addition of information to a file. The dictionary function: which permits search for information thanks to a code word or keyword The reading function: which allows all information placed on a magnetic record to be read.

Possible extensions:
. programmed learning, to be connected to an electric type-writer.

- The BRAILLINK III (3) from England (Clarke and Smith), with 45 Braille tactile characters. It uses magnetic tapes. It can interrogate data banks and search for information.

- The Braille devices with ephemeral characters from the electronic and technical Aids of MARBURG. These devices use Braille characters of 8 dots. The dot 7 represents a capital letter, the dot 8 indicates the position of the type-writer ball. It uses floppy discs. We have to mention the MBS 80 which has a memory of 2000 characters (25 lines of 80 characters), a complete screen. Two lines of 40 ephemeral characters allows us to read the Braille document.

- The BRAILLOCORD C(1) "Aid Electronic GMBH" Berlin, Germany:
with 32 Braille tactile characters. It has the possibility of searching for a word or a page and has a text editor.

- The VERSABRAILLE (12) Telesensory systems. U.S.A. With 20 ephemeral characters. It has the possibility for searching for chapters, blocks... It uses cassettes.

- The Microcassette (4) DATELEC Society, France with 20 ephemeral Braille characters and cassettes, it will be on sale by the end of this year. Note that its weight is only 900 grammes.

- The ORDIBRAILLE (6) from France, L.S.I. (Mr Patrick LIROU). It is a prototype of 20 ephemeral Braille characters. It will have different functions: text editor, dictionary function, reading function etc... and a program Braille 2 into Braille grade 1. Several manufacturers have been contacted and the decision have been will be taken at the end of this year.

For more information concerning the technical aids, you should consult the "International survey of aids for the visually disabled" published by John GILL.

V STANDARDIZATION OF SOFTWARE AND HARDWARE
Standardization of software:
In general a program written in FORTRAN language or in PASCAL language proves no problem for adaptation to a new computer or for their maintenance. The real problem is finding some spare time to undertake these modifications. May we hope a European Software Centre to remedy these availability problems?

Standardization of hardware:
It is "the problem". Even in Europe the code tables are not the same in many countries. We have therefore to put some modifications into our output files to use some devices.

As regards the device itself, real progress has been made for the interfaces: RS232C or V24 exist in many cases.

As regards cassettes or floppy disks we are all involved, program interfaces allow the exchange of records, but it is not easy and not generally available.

A big computer centre and networks make the communication and exchange of Braille files possible.

In addition to the previous standardization, I hope that the standardization of mathematics in Braille will be considered in the future. The mathematical language is a universal language in print, it is not the case in Braille. Various systems prevail in many countries, so a common code is desired in order to allow the blind scientific community to exchange documents.

CONCLUSION:
In spite of all the new devices which exist for the Blind (optical readers like OPTACON, synthetized voice etc...) the need for Braille remains. We know that when a blind person enjoys a talking book, his aim is to obtain that book in Braille-. We know that the blind who know Braille, require a Braille tactile output for the optical readers. But producing Braille documents necessitates expensive devices and staff. The blind community will not have all that exists for the sighted persons and the minimum of Braille we can produce them must be perfect:
Firstly, we hope that the Braille document will serve a pupil or a student.
Secondly, we hope that the number of readers increases year by year: The need for reading depends on the quality of the Braille. That was an observation made by Leslie CLARK, professor at Baruch College (New-York).
As regards the volume of Braille documents, one solution is the use of paperless devices or computers provided as a peripheral with a tactile board.
As for the programs, they bring many solutions relating to maintenance and the standardization.
The costs of upkeep up are often a burden for the users

18

and that will be eased in using software, not a special device.
    As regards standardization of the devices, I suppose that
it is difficult to find a solution acceptable to all the manufacturers. Why not focus our efforts on the VIDEO discs that
will perhaps resolve many problems when the Braille printing
houses want to exchange Braille documents.

REFERENCES:
DEBRAINE P. "L'avancement du system INSTIN-INJA" International
seminar "Computing and Braille" sept. 1981, TOULOUSE, FRANCE.
DUBUS J.P. "Dispositif autonome de traduction en Braille
intégral et abrégé" International seminar "computing and
Braille sept. 1981, TOULOUSE, FRANCE.
FRONTIN J. "Présentation d'un logiciel de transcription de la
musique en Braille". International seminar "computing and
Braille" sept. 1981, TOULOUSE, FRANCE. - "Présentation d'un
système pour la transcription de partitions musicales en
Braille" AFCET Congress, nov. 1981, GIF-SUR-YVETTE, FRANCE.
LIROU P. "L'ordibraille" International seminar "Computing and
Braille" sept. 1981, TOULOUSE, FRANCE.
MEEKEL J. "La transcription automatique des mathématiques en
Braille" AFCET Congress, nov. 1980, NANCY, FRANCE.
"Un système de production de textes mathématiques en Braille"
International seminar "computing and Braille" sept. 1981,
TOULOUSE, FRANCE.
"Un système de reconstitution de textes en écriture ordinaire à
partir de leur écriture Braille", Thèse de Docteur Ingénieur,
juin 1982, TOULOUSE, FRANCE.
"A system for transcribing mathematics into Braille" SIGCAPH -
Newsletter (ACM) 1983, N°31.
TRUQUET M. "The automatic transcription of French ink-print
into Braille" Research Bulletin, March 1974. - "Braille grade 2
Translator Program" - AFIPS 1976 - SIGCAPH ACM, N°20, 1976 -
"Braille at ROBIA Center" International Conference on
"Computerized Braille Production - TODAY and TOMORROW" - LONDON
- ENGLAND, May 1979.

ADDRESSES:
Aid Electronic GMBH Wilhelm von Siemens - Strasse 16/18 d -
1000 BERLIN 48.
BRAILLO NORWAY A.S. Brandsvei 5, p.o. box 647N - 3101 TONSBERG
- NORWAY.
CLARK AND SMITH Manufacturing Co Ltd Melbourne House, Melbourne
Road WALLINGTON, SURREY, ENGLAND.
DATELEC Society 2938, rue de l'Est 92200, BOULOGNE BILLANCOURT,
FRANCE.
Deutsche Blindenstudienanstalt Am Schalg 8D - 3550, MARBURG,
F.R.G.
L.S.I. (Laboratoire Langages et Systèmes Informatiques)
Université Paul Sabatier 118, route de Narbonne 31062, TOULOUSE
CEDEX, FRANCE.
LOUVAIN University (Pr FRANCOIS) Electronic Department
Kardinaal Mercierlaan 94B - 3030 LEUVEN, HEVERLEE, BELGIUM.
MARYLAND Computer Services 2010 Rock Spring Road Forest Hill,
MARYLAND 21050, USA.
PAPENMEIR-BRAILLEX Division p.o. BOX 1620D - 5840 SCHWERTE,
F.R.G.

PAPENMEIR-BRAILLEX Division p.o. BOX 1620D - 5840 SCHWERTE, F.R.G.
RESUS B.V. Wijnhaven 102 B 3011 WV ROTTERDAM, THE NETHERLANDS.
SAGEM Society, 6 avenue d'Iena 75783 PARIS CEDEX 13, FRANCE.
TELESENSORY Systems, Inc. 3408 Hillview Avenue PALO ALTO, CALIFORNIA, 94304, USA.
TRIFORMATION Systems, Inc. p.o. Box 2433 Stuart, FLORIDA 33494, USA.

PROGRESS IN AUTOMATIC PRODUCTION OF BRAILLE

H. Werner
Institut für Angewandte Mathematik
Rheinische Friedrich - Wilhelms - Universität
Wegelerstr. 6, D 5300 Bonn

Introduction

The problem of automatic Braille production by means of a computer has been with us for more than two decades. In fact the first informal meeting of scientists interested in automatic Braille production was organized during the IFIP congress 1962 at Munich. In the meantime a very fruitful cooperation took place between the European and the North – American countries. Today I am in the good position that Dr. Truquet, whose paper we just heard, has already defined the objectives, thus allowing me to launch into specific German problems. I am happy to report that we are leaving the experimental state of translation and setting up places for production. Emphasis is now layed on reducing the size of equipment needed for the translation process and putting it on a personal computer, which is even in the reach of institutions like schools or professionals. Though the programs became larger and larger, the personal computers grew so fast that they now can house such programs. The error quote of the transcription also is reduced so much that the result of automatic transcription depends mainly on the quality of the input. The daily inkprint newspapers show how bad this can be. With careful proofreading we can do much better.

Thus we can turn our attention to new tasks, perhaps not so spectacular as the general production but nevertheless important for some blind persons in order to become more independent in their professional work. In this respect we first turned to Braille code for mathematical publications. Unfortunately there are no international mathematical Braille standards up to date. Therefore we naturally use the rules established in Germany.

We can draw on development done by mathematicians in order to implement automatic typesetting of inkprint papers especially those with formulas. To non – mathematicians this task certainly looks difficult and indeed it took a considerable amount of work to create such an effective printing system. However the logical structure of a formula is easier to handle by means of computers than linguistic peculiarities as one meets them all along the production of literature in general.

The design of the general purpose translation programs.

The first version of a translation program from inkprint to contracted (Grad II) German Braille was written more than twenty years ago by students of mine and myself at Hamburg University and, later, Münster University. It was our objective, to produce a program that does not need any intervention during the translation. We were not willing to make any compromise in this respect. The first algorithm attacked the inkprint word letter by letter from left to right. Let us consider an example with an artifically shortened table of contractions.

Example of first algorithm

WELTGESUNDHEITSORGANISATION

W	WELCHER
	WER
	W
WE	WELCHER
	WER
	W
WEL	WELCHER
	WER
	W
WELT	WELCHER – not applicable
	WER – not applicable
	W (W) = $\begin{smallmatrix} o & o \\ o & o \\ o & o \end{smallmatrix}$

*ELTGESUNDHEITSORGANISATION

E	EL	
	ER	
	ES	
EL	EL	(EL) = $\begin{smallmatrix} o & o \\ o & o \\ o & o \end{smallmatrix}$
	ER	– not applicable
	ES	– not applicable

* * *TGESUNDHEITSORGANISATION

– – –

Reading the first letter i.e. W we test whether there is a contraction that can begin with this letter. If the answer is no, the letter is replaced by its Braille equivalent and the next letter is considered. This process allowed to cope with most of the rules even if it may not look like it at first sight. Take the case of the precedence rule. It says e.g. if the contraction 'es' 'or' 'ss' are colliding like in "Hesse", then the second and not the first contraction shall be used. This is handled by introducing an artificial contraction 'ess' und storing its correct translation '(e)(ss)` as a reference. (Here and in the following (e) refers to the Braille form that represents the letter e, etc.) The accuracy improved more and more by adding such artificial contractions to the table. But there seemed to be no end to it. The table was growing in no relation to the gain of accuracy.

Let me bring to your attention that the problems which seem to resist a formal logical analysis and hence programming are due to the fact that the application of Braille contractions is subjected to linguistic restrictions. Among other rules the contractions should not cross the border of the semantic fractures of a word. The German language possibly more than any other language allows for composite words. So there are many boundaries within words to be observed and many chances for wrong use of contractions. We learned from linguists that it is better to approach the splitting of a word into its components from its back than from its beginning i.e. not the way we read. It is even better to compare whole strings of letters simultaneously.

As a preparation for a new algorithm a big dictionary was to be set up, containing lists of letter strings and their correct Braille translation. Using the experience gathered with the first programs Professor Splett, some of his students, and some coworkers of our group compiled these lists with great effort. (We sometimes refer to them as Splett's rules.)

The result was a huge decision table which was run on a fairly big computer. For the sake of translation speed the most common German words were stored into a table called "file A" together with their Braille translations which provides for a quick access and transcription.

Unfortunately all words which are not in file A have to be scanned for all kinds of contractions and their possible translation. For this reason all possible contractions are stored for reference in a table called "file B".

In this new algorithm (Second Algorithm) the whole word as an entity has to be considered. The word is scanned for all contractions it contains by comparing with the entries of file B. If coincidence occurs the entry refers to an associated table showing those embedding letter strings in which the detected contraction needs special handling together with the proper transcription into Braille.

Let us demonstrate Splett's rules by considering the contraction 'richt' as an example. The first entry of the associated table is "aufricht". In this case the proper translation due to the semantics of the German language is the contraction for 'richt', because this string is probably part of the word "aufrichten" or a derivative of it. 'auf' is a prefix that can be contracted also.

The first seven entries contain the sylable 'richt' in the proper sense. In the next line it is not correct to use the contraction for 'richt' because "Trichter" has a completely different meaning. Thus in this case 'richt' is transcribed by the Braille form (r), the contraction for (ich) and the Braille form (t).

'richt' – table

– aufricht	(AUF)(RICHT)
– mitricht	(MIT)(RICHT
– zuricht	(ZU)(RICHT)
blutrichter	(B)(L)(U)(T)(RICHT)(ER)
kunstrichter	(K)(UN)(ST)(RICHT)(ER)
patentrichter	(P)(A)(T)(EN)(T)(RICHT)(ER)
stadtrichter	(ST)(A)(D)(T)(RICHT)(ER)
trichter	(T)(R)(ICH)(T)(ER)
kehricht	(K)(EH)(R)(ICH)(T)
röhricht	(R)(Ö)(H)(R)(ICH)(T)
töricht	((T)(Ö)(R)(ICH)(T)
mostricht	(M)(O)(ST)(R)(ICH)(T)
estricht	(E)(ST)(R)(ICH)(T)
– stricht	(ST)(R)(ICH)(T)
stricht	(ST)(R)(ICH)(T)
spricht	(S)(P)(R)(ICH)(T)
abricht	(A)(B)(RICH)(T)
bricht	(B)(R)(ICH)(T)
richt	(RICHT)

Continuing the translation process we delete the detected groups of letters step by step from the ink print input and procede with the rest of the word in the same way. (We also mark where the Braille text can be separated at the end of a line.) In this way translation is performed. Of course this lengthly search procedure consumes quite some time for going all over the inputted words. In producing this program we have applied certain tricks to get a reasonable speed of the translation but we will not discuss these technical details here.

We use the above example to show how a word is transcribed string by string.

Example of second algorithm

WELTGESUNDHEITSORGANISATION
1) ATION   WELTGESUNDHEITSORGANIS * * * * *
2) HEITS   WELTGESUND * * * * * ORGANIS * * * * *
3) NIS, IS WELTGESUND * * * * * ORGAN * * * * * * *
4) GES, (GE)WELT * * SUND * * * * * ORGAN * * * * * * *

5) UN   WELT**S**D*****ORGAN******
6) OR   WELT**S**D*******GAN*******
7) AN   WELT**S**D*******G*********
8) EL   W**T**S**D*******G*********

The final translation is

(W)(EL)(T)(GE)(S)(UN)(D)(HEIT)(S)(OR)(G)(AN)(IS)(ATION)

This example demonstrates how our current program works. In this process the size of the tables remains reasonable, but the searchtime rises considerably in spite of quite some programming effort. It fits, as said before, into the memory of microcomputers as they are sold as PCs ("personal computers") nowadays. These dedicated computers work not quite as fast as their big brothers, however, they are fast enough to meet the current demand, that is keep up with the input from the typists at the organisations and schools for the blind.

Braille Mathematics Code

After the good experience and success reached in automatic production of literature in grade II Braille we turned to special problems. As the first one we attacked the extension of the automatic translation to the production of mathematical Braille. Since there is no international standard so far, I hope that our attempt will produce a contribution that may help to path the way in the direction of standardisation. Although mathematical formulas can be understood by mathematicians world wide there is a variety of systems for transcribing them into Braille.

There are several problems to cope with. Two years ago I had the honour of participating in the promotion of Mr. Jaques Meekel under the supervision of Dr. Truquet at the University of Toulouse. He had designed a program system that allows him, the blind mathematician, to communicate not only with the computer but also with other mathematicians by producing an inkprint version of his paper typed in at a computer terminal. It was a difficult task to decode a Braille Mathematics Code and transcribe it to inkprint.

At Bonn University we attacked another problem. Starting from an inkprint math — ematical text, we wish to produce its Braille version. Because the technical problem of hardware is equal to that for ordinary Braille and since it can be considered satisfactorily solved we could concentrate on the software side:

        (i)   How do we input the text into the computer?

       (ii)   How should the text be written in Braille?

Let us first deal with the second problem.

In Germany the rules for writing Braille Mathematics Code had been studied and revised by a commission consisting of Dipl. Phys. Karl Britz, Professor Dr. Helmut Epheser, Dr. Gerrit van der Mey, and Dr. Friedrich Mittelsten – Scheid in 1955 and an extensive report edited by Professor Dr. Epheser was produced.

My student Pinell, himself blind, is thoroughly familiar with this German mathematical system. He is writing a computer program that will soon be available.

Let me briefly focus my attention at the difficulties we are facing in transcribing mathematical texts into Braille before I comment about its implementation.

Mathematical formulas as they appear in mathematical papers but also in many other sciences use a lot of different symbols in inkprint to denote the numerous entities that appear. To differentiate between them letters in different alphabets like Roman, Greek, Gothic, even Hebrew are used, it makes a difference whether they are small or capital letters and to increase the variety they are written slanted, cursive, bold face, script, sometimes with special little curles, to produce special symbols. These differences can be taken care of by prefixes introduced in Braille. Furthermore there are special symbols, like integrals and summation signs, and abbreviations that are international standard which are represented by corresponding symbols in Braille (Contractions). They are accompanied by certain rules about their possible positioning intended to avoid ambiguity or misunderstanding.

Some Braille symbols are marked to need an empty Braille cell ("space") on their left and/or right, others are marked to need a filled cell at the left and/or right and finally some are free in their composition with other symbols. Let me translate the corresponding German notions by "space needing", "space free" and "freely positionable".

The quoted report of Epheser formulates the following rules:

    i) There must not be an empty cell (space) between two symbols if (on the corresponding side) one of them is space free.

    ii) If neither of two neighboring cells is space free, but one is space needing, then an empty cell has to be inserted.

    iii) If both neighboring cells are freely positionable then an empty cell may optionally be inserted.

The properties "space needing" etc. are listed together with the meanings of the contractions. This is shown in the application to a small formula as an example using the following notations:

```
    ●● ○○ ○○ ●●
+   ●● ○○ ●● ●●
    ●● ○○ ●○ ●●

    ●● ○○ ○○ ●●
=   ●● ○○ ●● ●●
    ●● ○○ ●● ●●
```

```
                              ○○ ●●
                              ○● ●●
Prefix for small greek letter  ○● ●●
```

The full resp. empty Braille cells are used to indicate that + and = are space needing on the left and space free on the right side, the greek letter sign is space free on the right and freely positionable on the left. With these notations we may write:

```
○○ ●○ ○○ ○○ ●○ ○○ ○○ ●●
○● ○○ ○○ ●● ●○ ○○ ●● ○○
○● ○○ ○○ ●○ ○○ ○○ ●● ○○
   α       +   β       =   γ
```

It is obvious that these rules about the insertion of free cells are easily taken care of by a computer.

There are, however, instances as we will now see, when the empty cells have to be filled with special characters. You all know that mathematical formulas may contain exponents (upper indices) and they may also contain lower indices, (possibly not so common at schools). These indices may be composite expressions, they may even have their own additional indices. Generally speaking the inkprint layout may leave the current printing line and become two dimensional. In Braille one symbol follows the other one, thus we have to project everything on the current line. (Projection technique). This method is already used in inkprint to write fractions, occassionally. Ordinarily numerator and denominator are lifted up or pushed down, respectively. It is seen by the following example how this is handled in Braille.

ARABIC NUMBERS (with number sign
```
○●
○●
●●
```
)

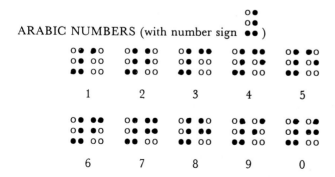

FRACTIONS (with fraction sign
●○
●●
○●)

```
            ○● ●○ ●○ ○● ●○                    ○● ●○ ○○
            ○● ○○ ●● ○● ●○                    ○● ○○ ●○
   1/2      ●● ○○ ○● ●● ○○   usually shortened ●● ○○ ●○
```

This shortened notation may be used if the numerator and denominator contains only numbers. The figures of the second number are shifted downwards within the Braille cell by one line. In general the projection is not quite as simple as for fractions but the clear structure of mathematical formulas nevertheless provides for clear production rules.

The line onto which the current text is written is called the "base line". In the German rules it is said that such a line is of rank one, two, etc. when it is reached by departing from the base line by one step, two steps, and so on. Necessary are of course means to denote the change from one rank to the other. This is either clear from a function, or it is explicitly specified by an operator for "upper index" or "lower index". Furthermore there are Braille codes which denote the rank which is entered or left. Counting is always done from the base line. Because there is the rule that there must not be an empty cell in any string that is not in the base line, empty cells are filled with the code for the current rank of these strings, as announced below. Instead of giving formal rules let me simply quote one example from Epheser.

In this example the following symbols are used

```
                        ○○ ●●                              ●● ○● ●●
                        ○○ ●●                              ●● ○○ ●●
small roman letter      ○● ●●         exponent             ●● ●● ●●

                        ○● ●●                              ○○ ●●
                        ○○ ●●                              ○● ●●
upper index             ●○ ●●         mark of base line    ○○ ●●

                        ●○ ●●                              ○● ●●
                        ○○ ●●                              ○○ ●●
lower index             ○● ●●         mark of first rank   ○○ ●●
```

PROJECTION TECHNIQUE (Epheser)

$$\left(x_n^i\right)^r$$

```
    ○○ ●● ●○ ●● ○● ○● ○● ●○
    ○○ ○○ ○○ ○● ○○ ●○ ○○ ●●
    ○● ●● ○● ●○ ●○ ○○ ●● ●○
```

$$\left(x_{n^i}\right)^r$$

```
    ○○ ●● ○○ ●○ ●● ○● ○● ○○ ○● ●○
    ○○ ○○ ○● ○○ ○● ○○ ●○ ○● ○○ ●●
    ○● ●● ○○ ○● ○○ ●○ ○○ ○○ ●● ●○
```

$$x_{n(i)^r}$$

```
    ○○ ●● ○○ ●○ ●● ○● ○● ○● ○● ●○
    ○○ ○○ ○● ○○ ○● ○○ ○○ ●○ ○○ ●●
    ○● ●● ○○ ○● ●○ ○○ ●○ ○○ ●● ●○
```

$$x_{(n^i)^r}$$

```
    ○○ ●● ○○ ●○ ●● ○● ○● ○● ●○
    ○○ ○○ ○● ○○ ○● ○○ ●○ ○○ ●●
    ○● ●● ○○ ○● ●○ ●○ ○○ ●● ●○
```

The marks of base line resp. ranks are used in this example to indicate how the letters are grouped. This is close to the mathematical way of using parentheses. It needs, as the computer scientist would say, "some book keeping" to do this organisation by computer, but from the design of compilers we have learned how to implement such a task.

We now return to the question of input of a mathematical text. The terminal of a computer is designed for sequential input, i.e. also in a projected way just as Braille print. Fortunately, in the last years mathematicians thought of meeting with the rising costs of mathematical typesetting by using computers for this purpose. There are now different operational systems available. One very advanced system called TEX was designed by Donald Knuth at Stanford University. It is now spread world wide at research institutions and universities, among others it has been adopted at our department at Bonn and augmented for the German language.

It just happens that this system is very well suited for transcription to mathematical Braille. Instead of lengthy explanations we repeat the above example and give its representation as TEX input together with the output produced by the computer.

$(x \sb n \sp i) \sp r$ $\left(x_n^i\right)^r$

$(x \sb {n \sp i}) \sp r$ $\left(x_{n^i}\right)^r$

$x \sb {n \sp {(i) \sp r}}$ $x_{n^{(i)^r}}$

$x \sb {(n \sp i) \sp r}$ $x_{(n^i)^r}$

Some notational remarks
$ denotes the beginning and end of mathematical expressions and formulas
sb   stands for subscript (lower index),
sp   for superscript (upper index),
the remaining symbols are self explanatory.

Mr. Pinell's program will use this type of input text and convert it into a Braille text. Since commercial users as printing houses start using TEX also for their publications it should be possible to obtain mathematical books and articles in Braille on demand just as easy as in inkprint. The structure of this input can be interpreted by processing from left to right using the cellar principle (in the language of computer scientists) and this means by the first algorithm which we saw in this paper. Hence processing of mathematical formulas shall be comparatively fast as compared to literary texts.

For the time being we have a number of texts that may serve for test purposes. It is hoped that the experience gathered in this way may help to improve and standardize the Braille mathematical code. In the meantime my coworkers and I are willing to look into some other fields of Braille applications. Hopefully we can report about this in not to far a future.

Literature

Jolley, Wm. Braille Mathematics Code – Prospects for a global approach.
  Braille International, Oct. 1981
Epheser, Helmut. Neufassung und Vervollständigung des Systems der internationalen Mathematikschrift für Blinde.
  Blindenstudienanstalt Marburg 1955
Raviv, Josef. Uses of Computers in Aiding the Disabled.
  Proceedings of the IFIP – IMIA working conference on uses of computers in aiding the disabled, Haifa 1981
  North – Holland Publishing Company, Amsterdam, New York, Oxford 1982
Splett, Jochen. Ein neues Verfahren zur automatischen Übersetzung in deutsche Blindenkurzschrift am Rechenzentrum der Universität Münster – linguistischer Teil.
  horus, Marburger Beiträge zum Blinden – Sehen, Heft 2, 10 – 13 (1979)
Werner, Helmut. Automatic Braille Production by Means of Computers.
  pp 321 – 336 in Raviv, J. (above quotation)
Werner, Helmut. Zwei Jahrzehnte automatische Herstellung deutscher Blindenschrift.
  Marburger Schriftenreihe zur Rehabilitation Blinder, Marburg 1984

AUTOMATIC PRODUCTION OF BRAILLE - A DANISH EXPERIENCE

P. Thomsen
Studiebogsbibliotek for Blinde (Students' Library)
Institute for the Blind
Copenhagen, Denmark

I THE EXISTING COMPUTERIZED BRAILLE PRODUCTION SYSTEM.

Since 1974 computer translation of inkprint material into grade 2
(contracted) Danish braille has been in operation.
The computerized translation and production procedures are:
  (i) Input
 (ii) Translation
(iii) Output
 (iv) Printing

INPUT

a. Editing; i.e. preparation of the inkprint text by a person
   familiar with braille and the braille code.
   After the necessary editorial decisions are made the inkprint
   material is handed over to a keypunch operator.
b. Transcription; the edited text is keyed character by character on
   punchcards (the punchcard-configuration) by an operator.
   During the keypunching the operator is responsible for the
   insertion of special braille editing codes indicating capitalization,
   numeral sign, italics and format controls like start new paragraph,
   force new line, force new page, tabulations, page numbers etc...

TRANSLATION

When the input is ready for processing the conversion of print to
braille is performed by computer.
A translation program and some tables ("The Dictionary") containing
the rules for the grade 2 braille system are loaded onto the computer
(IBM 370).
The translation program is designed to be table-driven rather than
being controlled by the program itself.
Because the program is table-driven a table switching mechanism is
included. The switching mechanism is able to handle the switching
from one braille system to another; e.g. grade 2 to grade 1, Danish
to German, Danish to English etc...
The translation program is not changed but only the pointers to the
tables, which gives the option within a text to switch from one
system to another.
The translation program operates at a speed of approxemately 8.000
words per minute.

OUTPUT

A magnetic tape resulting from the translation constitutes the
actual braille master.
The tape contains the different braille cells in form of codes and
the inkprint text which have generated the braille code.
A printout from the magnetic tape will not show the correct format
of a braille page. The formatting of the braille master is done
separately by use of a minicomputer PDP 11/10 before the actual
printing takes place.

PRINTING

A lineprinter, IBM 1403, with braille option, prints the final
braille book from the master.
The book is printed line by line at a speed of 420 braille lines
per minute or approxemately 20 braille pages per minute.
Except step one, input by punchcards, the other routines are still
the essential elements in the Danish computerized braille production
system.

II RENEWALS AND EXPERIMENTS

   (i) A substantial disadvantage of the described system was
       obviously the manual keypunching of the inkprint material.
       The procedure was found to be both time and cost consuming.
       The keypunching has therefore been replaced by a microcomputer
       system.
       The application of a microcomputer reduces both the entry time
       and improves the possibilities of a faster and more flexible
       way of correcting and editing the text.
       However, a manual transcription of the inkprint material is still
       necessary before an automatic and faster translation and printing
       into braille can take place.
  (ii) A more direct access to printed material and with a minimum of
       human intervention seems possible by applying compositors or
       photocomposition tapes used in the printing industry for
       production of inkprint texts.
       If the text is available in machine-readable form on a magnetic
       or papertape for composition of inkprint it is already
       demonstrated feasible to use the composition tape as an input
       to a computer translation into braille.
       One of the main problems however, in the application of
       compositors tapes for braille production is that the tapes are
       provided with various composition codes for the inkprint setting
       Most of these codes are useless in braille (e.g. bold-face,
       petit, italics, type size, page format, etc...). They have to
       be identified and removed or transformed before the tape can
       serve as an input to computerized braille production.
       However, this process - "cleaning" - can be accomplished by a
       special computer interface program - a preprocessor.
       In Denmark we have experimented with texts on machine-readable
       form from the following sources:
       a. The Regional Computer Centre of the University of Copenhagen
          (RECKU);

b. a publishing house (Gyldendal)
c. a central data bank of a publisher (Schultz)

RECKU

RECKU produces university magazines, periodicals, reports etc...
from photocomposition tapes.
It has proved relatively uncomplicated to produce braille texts
from the same tapes. This is because the text and most of the
type-setting or composition codes are kept separately on special
lines, on the tape. Consequently, the superflous codes can easily
be removed from the tape and it becomes rather simple to write a
preprocessor for the cleaning of the actual text.

GYLDENDAL

The texts used from "Gyldendal" are novels and short stories.
The composition codes and commands, in this case, are found
both in text and on separate lines; thus making the preprocessor
programming much more complicated.
Not only that you have to remove the codes which are entered
separately, but you also have to search the text itself for
composition codes. We have, however, reached a stage where it
possible to use the compositors tapes from "Gyldendal" as the
basic entry source for the production of books in braille.

SCHULTZ

The "Schultz" publishing house is the greatest publisher of law
books, laws, official reports of parliamentary proceedings and
the like.
The material is kept in machine-readable form and kept in a central
data bank.
The main problem in producing braille from the "Schultz" compositors
tapes is the lay-out of the texts, more than the "cleaning" and the
translation of the text itself.
In addition to both ordinary and special composition codes (paragraph,
subsection, number) you have many more editorial control codes than
for ordinary texts.
Most of the composition codes and the editorial ones cannot be
translated automatically into equivalent braille codes.
The Danish experience, so far, is that such texts and for textbooks
in general, the required lay-out in print as in braille is the
greatest obstacle for an automatic production from compositors
tapes.
In order to produce a satisfactory brailly copy of the "Schultz"-
texts and simular ones a great deal of human intervention has
been required.
A person familiar with the Danish braille code and braille formatting
and lay-out tapes in, via a microcomputer, the necessary braille
editorial control codes before the text is translated and printed.
The experiences with use of compositors tapes and automatic
production of braille have exposed two (2) other substantial
problems.

(i) There is, up to now, very little standardization of composition codes within the publishing industry. This situation results in the need for elaboration of an interface program - a preprocessor - for each publisher whose compositors tapes you get access to.

(ii) In Danish there is a conflict between the braille code and the contraction of a number of Danish compound words in relation with automatic translation of print to braille. In Danish the letter combinations sk-, st-, ing- and ng- are very common. Therefore they are represented in the Danish braille code by a one-cell contraction and are given priority to any other contraction possibility.
Examples: huSKe (remember)
          heSTe (horses)
          peNGe (money)
          brINGe (to bring)
In the following compound words the same contraction possibilities appear, but should never be used.
Examples: hus/kat (house cat)
          hus/tag (roof)
          maskin/gevær (machine gun)
In an automatic translation of print to braille the computer cannot distinguish between simple words and compound words; thus using the contractions SK in "hus/kat", ST in "hus/tag" and ING in "maskin/gevær".
In order to produce an error-free braille text it is therefore necessary to scrutinize the text for all compound words and insert a hyphenation mark for each word.
Without the human intervention it is possible to produce a 99% correct braille edition which has been accepted by blind people depending on a fast access to printed material for their work.
Likewise, many employed people do have access to printed material in machine readable form, so if they accept the few contraction errors we can offer them an almost automatic translation into braille.
On the other hand, it is obvious, that for books for the braille library, they must be in a perfect grade 2 Danish braille.

III FUTURE DEVELOPMENT AND EXPERIMENTS

(i) In order to reduce further the described manual intervention it is planned to work out an editorial program which automatically can search the text for compound problem words.
One way to identify the problem words could be to provide the program with a listing of all such words.
Once the word is identified the program should automatically insert a hyphenation mark.
This routine is supposed to take place prior to the preprocessing and translation.

(ii) Some of the major publishers in Denmark contemplate offering writers and translators microcomputers and word-processing systems.

In that case the basic material for the braille production
could be a discette with the "raw" text free of composition
and typesetting codes instead of a compositor tape.
Consequently the discette would not have to be "cleaned"
before it can be used for braille production.
A further perspective is that the publishers do envisage
using the same computer systems and programs; thus reducing
the need of having one specific preprocessing program for
each publisher.
However, before any access to such discettes might be granted
there must be an amendment of the Danish copyright law.
To-day we have a free access to all printed material for
transcription into braille.
Before we can start using text-carrying discettes or compositors
tapes for braille production on a regular basic a solution to
the copyright question must be found.

(iii) A further extension of the existing production system should
be the use of optical reading via an Kurzweil data-entry-
system. The actual ocr-reading would be done by a service
bureau in possesion of a Kurzweil multi-font reading machine.

(iv) The major task of the Danish Printing House for the Blind
is to mass-produce magazines and periodicals.
The printing house still uses the conventional manual
stereotyping equipment for that purpose. In the future the
manual stereotyping equipment will be replaced by an
electronic stereotyping system including editorial and
proofreading facilities. With the existing computer equipment
it is possible to run a small scale production system as
well as a system for large editions.

IV AUTOMATIC PRODUCTION OF TEXTBOOKS.

The problems involved in an automatic production of textbooks from
compositors tapes have already been touched previously in this paper.
The blind person must be presented with the same information content
as his sighted peers in a normal printed book and as far as possible
in the same consecutive form and in an equivalent lay-out.
This is essential for blind people working together with sighted
people and for students in an integrated educational situation.
Otherwise it risks excluding a mutual communication. For these
reasons the inkprinted book must be revised before it is transcribed
into braille. In the case of textbooks this revision is extremely
costly and often time-consuming. The revision should be carried
out by a specialist.
Furthermore, the transcription of many textbooks requires the
use of special braille notation systems and the elaboration of
tactile graphical material. Likewise, tables and listings requires
a thorough revision before they can be transcribed into braille.
As however there is no or at least very few textbooks without
long passages of continous prose it should be feasible to fit
such passages of continous text into an automatic braille production
system.
At the Students' Library at the Institute for the Blind in Copenhagen,
Denmark, we have no such experiences yet.

Our future plans are to make use of existing compositors tapes for textbooks and to make the required revision via a microcomputer system. The versatility of the "RECKU" text-editing system makes it already possible to work out a complete list of the 63 braille signs which can be displayed on a crt-screen.

With the application of such a text-editing system the specialist would perform the necessary revision of complicated passages at the "braille"-screen and then enter them directly to the text-carrying medium (e.g. compositors tapes or discettes).

V CONCLUSION

The Danish experiences as well as current research in other countries indicate so far that a future computerized braille production based on compositors tapes might result in:

   (i) shorter production time; in principle it should be technical
       feasible to publish the braille edition at the same time as
       the inkprint one;
  (ii) considerable extension of the access to printed material
       for blind people;
 (iii) possibility of continous up-dating of braille texts printed
       from compositors tapes;
  (iv) flexibility in the choice of format.

Production experience over a longer period of time will be required before these advantages can be determined and quantified.

INNOVATION, BRAILLE INFORMATION AND WORKPLACE DESIGN
M. SOEDE

Institute for Rehabilitatioon Research
Zandbergsweg 111, 6432 CC Hoensbroek - THE NETHERLANDS

INTRODUCTION
Developments in our society create new problems for the handicapped. Especially for the blind, the gap between non-handicapped and handicapped could increase due to the following developments: New jobs and tasks in the field of technology and information involve higher demands and are often more and more specialized. Partly due to this and also due to economic problems, the high unemployment rates affect the situation of the handicapped more than others. Instead of normal jobs, work at home, including free-time allocation and recreation, will become more important.

Finally, preparation for new specialized jobs involves a strong emphasis on education and study by the handicapped person. The blind person's concern is to keep up his possibilities as well as he can by using Braille and other oppurtunities for communication and information handling.

GOALS
The main goal is to reduce or to prevent an enlargement of the gap which exists between oppurtunities for handicapped and non-handicapped persons. More specifically this will mean for the blind and visually impaired that:
- Aids have to be developed which adapt working situations so that they can be used by the blind, or which will give some compensation. The exchange of those task elements which cannot be handled by the blind and visually impaired with non-handicapped colleagues might be one example.
- More jobs and occupations have to be explored for handicapped persons. Much attention is focused on "typical" jobs for the blind, but especially in the field of information technology, new jobs/ occupations are becoming available, and these should be carefully considered by the visually impaired person.
- Technological development has to be guided in a more "handicap-friendly" direction and/or alternatives and options in the uses for modern equipment have to be incorporated into this equipment.

ASPECTS OF THE PRESENT SITUATION
It is expected that office work will comprise more than 50% of jobs in the near future. Within these jobs there will be about 40-60% of tasks which deal with information handling activities. These activities include reading, writing, keyboard operation, computer file operations and many others. Due to the important role of the computer, the number of terminals will increase from one terminal for 25 people to 1:7 in the near future and, eventually, a ratio of 1:3 could be expected.

Besides the important role of keyboard/terminal activities in professional situations, the use of keyboards will also increase in hobby and daily tasks such as banking and shopping. A new information display technology, automatic speech production, could have an important impact for the visually impaired. However, at this moment, the quality is far from sufficient to use in a text reading machine situation. And for applications in computer tasks it is not yet very well understood how it should be used: Not enough human factor knowledge on this subject is available.

Also the tactile information transfer in the case of large Braille displays and full page graphic displays is not very well understood from the ergonomic viewpoint. Nevertheless it will be a great opportunity if such display systems become commercially available.

A very serious aspect in the evolution of computer technology from the viewpoint of the visual impaired person is that terminals are optimized in the direction of the use of visual information. This can be illustrated by the following examples:

- Touch panels/displays which are programmed as a display screen represented to control the execution of programs cannot be used in this way by the visually impaired.
- The same can be said of the "mouse"-control and, in general, all cursor control devices which are based on display screen oriented software menu's.
- Software is developed with a strong emphasis on the lay-out on the screen: the lay-out itself includes a lot of information. Examples are the "spread-sheet"-systems, vision software and menu-systems as used in the IBM-PC and the MacIntoch personal computer.
- Terminals of larger computer systems transfer the information from and to the computer by a video-signal. The consequence is that it is difficult to connect a parallel braille-system to the terminal.

These software and hardware developments are in favour of the sighted user. To change such a development will be impossible but more possibilities for less screen-oriented systems connected in parallel, have to be considered.

Finally, from a small survey project in the Netherlands on employment aspects of visually impaired persons it is seen that the blind employees in offices consider automatization as a threat to their position and not as a challenge providing new possibilities which could be explored by them.

SOME CONSIDERATIONS ON WORKPLACE DESIGN

Physical/environmental aspects: A large amount of literature is available on the physical aspects of workplace design for non-handicapped office workers. This literature deals with illumination, temperature, environmental noise, seating, arrangement of office furniture, administrative equipment, etc. Almost no literature is available about these aspects dealing with the special influence on a handicapped person. For the blind office employee it is necessary to draw attention to: Seating and posture in relation to desk-height. An essential difference with the non-handicapped person is the reading process. Braille reading requires enough flat space on a table and a height of the table which is comfortable for a good hand position for the tactile reading process. A recommendation is to have as a table height a reading surface which is about 5cm

lower than normal table heights (most tables for typists will be of a proper height).
Position of hardware elements. The proper place of hardware elements has to be found such that the elements (cassette recorder, dictating machine, telephone, keyboards, etc.) can be located by touch without actual searching.
Document filing. High stacks of documents are most inconvenient to handle for blind people. It is therefore necessary to provide enough space like additional benches, large tables and drawers to prevent the piling up of documents as much as possible.
Hardware ergonomics, input devices: Using braille information imposes a different human factor design of the input equipment. While the hands are used for reading as well as for input of data there has to be either a sequential action pattern or a one-hand reading and one-hand keyboard operation. A user selectable software conversion of the two-hand 8-dot Braille keyboard to a one-hand operated keyboard would be a solution.

The use of normal type keyboards poses the problem of having little standardization of key configuration; most of the characters are equally located in most systems, but large variations occur in the arrangement of operation and function keys.

From a practical viewpoint it strongly inhibits the blind person getting used to the several available keyboards in an office environment.

In addition to the problem of various arrangements, there is also lacking a normalization of translation of operation keys and function keys in a Braille code: each manufacturer solves this in his own way. This is not just an additional burden to the blind employee, who has to work with more than one keyboard system, but it also causes severe trouble if input data comes from other sources like Viditel and Teletex data banks.

Furthermore, it has to be recommended that the frequently available numeric key pad should have an arrangement which is the same as the telephone touch pad.

Finally, it is expected that speech recognition will be a user-friendly manner of entering data to computer systems. Until now, it seen that the available recognition systems are not sufficiently accurate for use in text and data processing. Brochures of manufacturers claim recognition rate of 99% with vocabularies of 100-200 words. Reports on current experience, however, show recognition rates of 85 to 90%.
Hardware ergonomics, output devices: A variety of Braille printing machines are commercially available. The quality of print, the speed and the price of these machines cover broad ranges. There is not yet quite a good understanding of the relationship between printed Braille and paperless Braille. Blind people report having a great need for larger paperless Braille displays (page size) and graphics displays.
Unfortunately, there is almost no research done which either confirms or denies the usefulness of large displays. Product development institutes and manufacturers are therefore very reluctant to be involved in the design and production of such displays.

Finally, it is of major importance for a blind employee that his Braille oriented workplace will also provided with a visual display unit and/or an ink-print machine. This is needed for communication with colleagues and the take over of tasks in case of absenteeism.

Software ergonomics: In an office workplace based on Braille information there will be several software modules applicable. Depending on tasks, function, experience, etc., a selection has to be made from one of the following modules:
- instruction manual
- file manipulator
- code transformation: Braille to ASCII and vice-versa
- system control
- text editor/word processor
- archive/library system
- memo pad/scratch pad
- agenda
- directories
- special software to be developed or bought for special applications and adapted in order to be used by blind persons.

Most of the software is commercially avialable but requires, in most cases, a very costly adaption for use by the blind.

With respect to this aspect one has to select a proper man-machine dialogue form. Five basic possibilities for the dialogue are given in Table 1, below.

Menu selection and Blank form are visual display screen oriented: a particular position on a screen has to be indicated or, respectively, has be selected. These systems are quite unsuitable for the blind.

Table 1: Man-machine dialogue forms

Type	Suitability for use by the blind
Menu selection	-
Blank form	-
Command lay-out example	+
Parametric commands	+
Natural language	0

Command lay-out example and Parametric commands require a string of text not related to a position on (an optional) screen; the string is like a previously given example or, respectively, appears as a number of parameter values which denote special program options. These systems are suitable for the blind but involve an extended training period: particularly the parametric command method requires much memorizing.

The natural language is not available at a commercial level for a reasonable price, but might be a very interesting method if it becomes fast enough and cheap enough.

Design of an individual workplace: The design of a individual workplace for the blind can best be done by taking three steps as follows:
- Analysis of the job and specific tasks that have to be performed by the blind employee.

- A selection of the appropriate hardware elements and software elements which have to be based on the analysis as mentioned.

- An adaptation of the hardware and software to suit the individual workplace and to evaluate performance afterwards.

To illustrate the individuality of this process two tables are given (adapted from: H.K. Boswijk, 1982: See the list of references). In the first table (Table 2) it can be seen that workplace equipment is related to information handling activities.

The second table (Table 3) presents some examples of office functions in relation to information processes and type of information.

Whereas these tables are applicable for non-handicapped persons, a conversion has to be made in case of a blind employee: different equipment solutions and different accents on information handling are coming up. Furthermore, it happens rather often that tasks are exchanged between jobs, such that a particular job becomes more suitable for a blind person. It is recommmended that more research should be done with respect to job analysis in relation to special equipment selection to aid the visually impaired.

Table 2: Equipment and information handling activities

equipment \ information processes	generation	transformation	indexing	storage & retrieval	selection	transmission	multiplication	presentation	destruction
dictating machine			o			o			
telephone						o	o		
typewriter			o			o	o		
text processing	o		o	o		o	o		
teletext	o	o		o		o	o	o	
copying machine							o	o	
computer terminal	o	o	o	o				o	o
viditel				o	o			o	
microfiche reader			o	o				o	
personal computer	o	o							
multifunctional terminal	o	o	o	o	o	o	o	o	o

Table 3: Jobs and information aspects

jobs	generation	transformation	indexing	storage & retrieval	selection	transmission	multiplication	presentation	destruction	interpretation	text	data	graphical	audio	visual
manager	o					o	o				o	o	o	o	o
secretary		o	o				o	o	o		o	o		o	
bookkeeper	o	o	o			o			o		o	o	o		
archivist			o	o	o	o			o		o	o	o		
personnel official	o	o				o				o	o	o		o	o
salesman	o	o				o				o	o	o		o	o
researcher	o	o		o	o	o				o	o	o	o	o	o

CONCLUSIONS: MODULAR APPROACH NEEDED

From the above mentioned paragraphs a major conclusion can be drawn: equipment for the visually impaired has to be developed as functional modules based on "standard" commercially available equipment. More reasons for this are:
- Dedicated equipment is aiming at compromise solutions. These solutions are mostly rather conventional in order to try to obtain a large share of the market, and not optimal in a specific workplace or perofession.
- Commercial "standard"; equipment with adaptations for special use by the blind will frequently make use of software delivered with this equipment. Manufacturers of consumer goods plan far ahead in technology.

Thus, it is not advisable to develop any further specialized complete Braille terminals.

Attention has to be drawn to the development and adaptation of low-cost functional components.

Finally, this type of development has to be accompagnied by organizational measures in order to provide proper assistance in selection, adaptation and installation of modules in a workplace.

REFERENCES

Boswijk, H.K.; Informatie en communicatie voor het kantoor in de toekomst. (Information and communication in the office of the future). In: Het kantoor van de toekomst: de toekomst van het kantoor. Nixdorf Computer B.V., Utrecht, 1982.

Crenshaw, J.W., Philipose, J. Can computers really be friendly? Computer Design, Feb. 1983, pp. 103 - 108.

Gould, J.D. Composing letters with computer-based text editors. Human Factors, 1981, 23 (5), pp. 593 - 606.

Liebelt, L.S., McDonald, J.E., Stone, J.D., Karat, J. The effect of organization on learning menu access. Proc. of Human Factors Soc. 26th Annual Meeting, 1982, pp. 546 - 550.

Ogden, W.C., Boyle, J.M.; Evaluating Human-Computer Dialog Styles: Command VS. Form/Fill-in for report modification. Proc. of Human Factors Society, 26th Annual Meeting, 1982, pp. 542 - 545.

Scapin, D.L.; Computers commands in restricted natural
language: Some aspects of memory and experience. Human
Factors, 1981, 23 (3), pp. 365 - 375.

Schalk, T.B., Van Meir, E.L.; Terminals , listen up , speech
recognition is a reality. Computer Design, sept. 1983.
(97 - 102).

Soede, M.; Innovation in aids for the handicapped; some
critical remarks on automatic speech technology. Proc.
Workshop on communication, Oct. 19 - 21, 1983 , Göteborg,
11 p.

Soede, M., Raaymakers, E.M.J.A. Een Werkplek computer voor
blinden; aanbevelingen specificaties. (A workplace computer
for the blind; recommendations for specifications).
RESUS - Rotterdam B.V./Neth. Inst. for Prev. Healthcare -
Leiden, 1982, internal report, 86 p. (in Dutch).

Williams, R.D. A systems analysis approach to office
automation. Proc. of Human Factors Society, 26th Annual
Meeting, 1982, pp. 302 - 306.

Projectgroep Zintuiglijk en Orgaan Gehandicapten. Technolo-
gische innovatie ten behoeve van zintuiglijk en orgaan gehandicapten (Project group sensory and organically impaired.
Technological innovation for the sensory and organically
impaired), The Hague/Leiden. First and second report. Min. of
Science and Education. 1980/1981.

NECESSARY PRIORITY AREAS IN THE DEVELOPMENT OF TECHNICAL AIDS FOR THE BLIND IN THE FEDERAL REPUBLIC OF GERMANY

M. HARRES

Deutsche Blindenstudiesnanstalt
Am Schlag 8, Postfach 11 60
D-3550 Marburg/Lahn

In the second half of the 70's the Federal Government carried out a priority study, the aim of which was to develop new technical aids for the blind, right up to the stage of series production. This priority study was supported and sponsored financially by private institutions. During this period the following developments were made:
- tactile lines
- Braille recorders and
- machines to rationalize the process of book printing for the blind.

The Government also financed a study to investigate the numer of technical aids in use by the blind, and to establish the age range among the blind, as well as their degree of education and general knowledge. The development of a reading machine with Braille and speech output was implemented but unfortunately abandoned after being promoted over a period of three years. I do not wish to go into the individual products which were developed to the production stage during this period of time. I shall take it that most of you are sufficiently familiar with them. The aim of the priority study - to improve integration of the blind in the professional and vocational sphere - has, in our view, been successfully achieved. Many jobs and apprenticeships depend today on these devices and are completely unthinkable without these new devices. But much as this development and priority by technological change. Some of these devices are, in my opinion, already outdated and are only being used for want of something better.

In many cases today they are, in fact, an impediment to the integration of the handicapped, because, for example, they may be incompatible with each other, or because the process of connecting them up to commercial systems is an extremely complicated one. Another point is that the systems promoted by the Government and in production today do not allow for direct access to stored texts, whether in book form or to data bases in central computers, in data banks or on video texts. The difficulties involved in recalling stored data arise from the problems of text input for all kinds of ink-print texts, and of reproducing data from data banks.

First, I should like to go into text input for ink-print texts. The ideal machine for the input of printed text is still the reading machine with an unlimited range of symbols, or 'Multifont'. As I have already mentioned, this development, as part of the priority study, was shelved.

Basically, a reading machine must fulfil the following requirements. Firstly, the rate of reading mistakes must be reduced to a minimum. Then, the blind must be given certain possibilities of interaction. Let me explain this in more detail. The written material which a blind person feeds into a reading machine is, both from the point of view of content and structure, unknown to him at the outset i.e. the material can be of various type sizes, the texts can be written in columns, there can be illustrations in the text etc. The letter size can vary greatly within the text. Furthemore, the process of reading can be interrupted by drawings, pictures or text passages written in columns. It is therefore necessary to give the blind reader a tactile presentation of the reading material before he starts to read the text. The intention of such a tactile presentation of the written material is to give the blind reader a general impression, an overall view, of the form and structure of the text. It should enable him to recognize where pictures, for example, have been added to the text or what size of type has been used, or whether the text has been divided into columns. The overall impression he gains from this tactile presentation should be comparable to the impression a sighted person has of the form of a text from a distance of about 10 metres. From this distance the sighted reader can see what the structure of the text is. With the help of this tactile presentation, the blind user could programme the machine onto the requisite graphic tablet by feeding in the size of print to be read, and by giving instructions as to the order in which the text should be read and as to which sections are to be read. Such a presentation of the text which is to be read could be transmitted to the blind reader by means of a whole-page display, with a distance between the dots of approximately 2,5 to 2,7mm horizontally and vertically - this corresponds approximately to the distance between the dots in large-size Braille print. This whole-page display could then fulfil three functions:

1. it could give a tactile presentation of the structure of the text

2. it could take over the functin of a graphic tablet and

3. it could present the text, which has been read, in Braille.

At present there is a reading machine for sighted people on the world market, which can also be used as the basis of a reading machine for the blind - the Kurzweill reading machine. If we leave out the question of price, which amounts to about 220.000,--DM for this machine, the use of such a machine would be extremely worthwhile for the blind in the field of work. The price, however, does not favour such use. Such a machine could also be used in the field of Braille printing to feed in texts in print; other places which would benefit from its use would be big libraries, which store books for the blind in data carriers, which can then be recalled by the blind user in his Braille reproduction device. One could also imagine that the data of a stored ink-print book could then be played to the blind by telephone.

I should now like to turn to the recall of data from data bases eg. central computers, data banks or video texts. The data are structured in such a way they can be presented on

video screens. This means that the data - before they can be presented to a blind person - must be adapted to suit the purposes of the blind. The type of adaptation depends on the medium used for output. Today there are only 2 basic possibilities for output:
- tactile presentation in Braille, either on paper or on tactile lines and
- speech output.

Firstly, I should like to deal with speech output. Text output in synthetic language is really only suitable for short texts and text controls. This should only be used in jobs which entail a high degree of decision-making. That means for jobs which, because of the brevity of the information transmitted to person responsible, call for qualified handling of this information. This would apply in the case eg. of programmers or of personnel in accountancy and bookkeeping. It seems to me that speech output would not be suitable for studying academic texts, neither in schools nor at university. Nor can I imagine tha the blind would accept this synthetic language for the presentation of aesthetic literature.

The fact that 43% of the visually handicapped, given the choice, would opt for this artificial speech output and not for Braille as a means of transmitting information would appear to contradict this. At present, however, there is no speech output in German which is based on the German phonetic system and which does justice not only to the sentence melody but also to the word melody which is essential if it is to sound pleasant. Some firms have made developments which run on large computers and which therefore achieve the aim of producing an acceptable quality of speech.

As far as the study and the reading of longer texts is concerned, Braille output is, in my opinion, still the best medium for the blind. Here, we heve several possibilities.

Firstly, embossing onto paper. The main disadvantage of embossing on paper is the embossing speed; and embossing is very expensive, because on the one hand the available Braille machines are very expensive and, on the other, a great deal of paper is produced. A further disadvantage of Braille-output is the change of format which results with output.

The texts which are stored in data bases are, as I've already mentioned, prepared for presentation on TV screens. This presentation often contains essential information for the sighted which is lost to the blind user because of the change of format involved using Braille output. In some instances this information can be transmitted to the blind by delivering the texts on tactile lines which have been adapted to match the screen size. I am thinking here of a double row of 2 X 40 symbols. And yet, the essential overall view of the individual parts of the data presented is lost to the blind user. Furthemore, there is the difficulty of reading columns of numbers.

The following are missing with data output structured for video screens - the whole-page display, and a reasonably-priced printer, which would be used when required to imprint the information. Both devices, the whole-page display and the inexpensive printing device, would have to be constructed so that they could be connected to the standard interface of any video-screen. In addition, it should be possible to present graphics with both machines. This would be possible if both machines were constructed to work with a distance between the dots of 2.5mm horizontally and vertically (in directions X and Y). It goes without saying that both machines would have to be reasonably-priced and safety-tested.

Allow me to summarize what I have already said.

We have four priority areas in need of development:

1. The reading machine with Multifont and a graphic tablet for the blind.

2. The whole-page display with a distance between dots of 2.5mm.

3. The inexpensive printing machine, which can also produce graphics.

4. Speech output, based on a German set of phonetics.

Let me return once again, finally, to the study I mentioned, which was carried out by the Government within the framework of the priority study. As part of this study the age range of the blind was investigated. It became clear that 68% of all blind people are over 60. The total number of blind people in the Federal Republic amounts to approximately 75,000 at present; that is around 1.2%. Of these 75,000 only 15,000 are able to read Braille, and only 13% of the total number of the blind work and 3% are still to complete their education or training. The necessary aids compiled by me are therefore only of use to a small minority of the blind. This study also showed that the number of elderly blind familiar with the technical aids on offer is very small indeed. Only about 37% of the total amount of visually handicapped persons and 18% of the elderly blind are aware of the existence of technical aids on offer or know about the German Aid Centres. For this reason I consider another priority area to be absolutely essential for the coming year: in my opinion we must undertake measures directed at publicising and making people aware of the availability of technical aids.

At the moment in the Federal Republic of Germany there is little hope of completing the necessary developments. On the one hand, the Government has already distributed the available funds elsewhere — for the promotion of priority areas for other handicapped groups; at the moment, for example, they are sponsoring technical aids for the deaf and hard of hearing. Furthermore, the independent Boards and institutions for the blind have less money at their disposal than was the case a few years ago. I therefore see only two possibilities for developments to make at least partial headway. Firstly, we shall be forced to annex ourselves to commercial developments; this would be possible with the development of synthetic language and with the construction and use of reading machines for the blind. Secondly, I consider close European cooperation to be absolutely necessary in order to make effective use of the available funds.

DISCUSSION

Werner (to Soede)

How much could you take from commercial systems in the implementation of your workplace?

Soede

I fear that not so much can be used from commercial systems without any change. But I think that a lot of programs are available
and can be adapted rather easily to be used in the field of data
handling, file manipulation, text editing. The man/machine communication has to be completely different even in those cases
where basic software modules can be used. This is not difficult
because modern systems handle so easily peripheral equipment.

Soede (to Werner)

I was wondering this morning why the Braille translation problem
doesn't use the knowledge that is developed for the production
of speech systems. The advanced speech systems are based on a lot
of knowledge about language. It is basically a coding and an understanding problem, for example, how to lay an accent in a sentence. That type of knowledge should be useful for translating
texts into Braille.

Werner

The method of translating inkprint into Braille seems to be completely different from the way you are splitting the output of
speech. As far as I can see there is no relationship we could
really use. In fact, we have designed speech output software at
the University of Münster and we have gathered some experience in
this direction. Also other systems are being produced in Bochum
by colleagues in electroengineering. The problem in our translation program is the linguistic part. To achieve the high accuracy
we have obtained now we had to look at every single word. Perhaps
it didn't come out clearly enough in my lecture this morning how
much manpower has been invested in this linguistic work. It is
difficult for me to estimate it, but I think 20 years of manpower is a fair estimate because we had quite a number of persons
involved, screening, searching, scanning all the words and keeping track of any corrections that are needed for the Braille
translation. The analogy between speech output and written output
as it is coded nowadays in our formalized languages seems only
rather superficial, I feel.

Truquet

Also for French, we have many problems. We cannot use what is
made for synthesized voice. I tried to work with a team which is
preparing a big dictionary for synthetic voice. But it was not

possible to output at the same time the voice and the Braille, because French is phonetic and grammatical. So when it is not phonetic we have to go for the rules and the dictionary.

Emiliani (to Thomsen)

I would like to ask a question about the translation from compositor tapes into Braille. How could you solve the problem of copyright? I would also like to know from other people in other nations, if in their country it was possible to cope with this problem. In Italy we were not able, up to now, to obtain the permission to use compositor tapes for the reproduction with Braille.

Thomsen

The problem of copyright for the use of compositor tapes has not been solved by us so far. There must be an amendment, a change in the Danish copyright law before we can start producing Braille from compositor tapes on a regular basis. So far, this activity has only been carried out on an experimental basis. The problem is that, once you have these compositor tapes, clean or with type setting codes, you can produce anything from it.

Werner

We have been using linotype tapes for not quite 20 years, I think, since 1968. But we were in direct cooperation with the printing houses that produced them because the output in inkprint and in Braille appears just parallel, to achieve a regular edition of a bi-weekly Braille newspaper (Zeit-Stern Magazin). So, we didn't have any of these problems and, so far, in the experimental stage, the printing houses would grant us the right to use the tapes. Otherwise, I think, it's just a problem to be resolved by the institutions, and not the technicians.

François

The editors we have contacted in Belgium have shown no problem concerning copyrights. Instead, the ones we have contacted said: "It's a great honour for us that you want to transcribe our books in Braille, and you are quite welcome to come to our offices, and we will help you to put them on your computer. You are welcome any time".

Thomsen

In Denmark, the situation may be a little bit different because the copyright holder is not the editor, but the writer.

Emiliani

I think it is different if you have to produce a newspaper or a book because, obviously, for the newspaper, you don't have the

problem of reproduction. You don't have the problem that someone else wants to reproduce the today's newspaper after one week.
With books, it is completely different. I think that this is a
very important problem and, probably, it should be studied on a
European scale.

Levett (to Mandar)

I think the problem of searching, detecting, recognizing, is a
very important general problem, that we can recognize in the visual system or in the tactile system or any neurophysiological
system, as well as man-made systems with targeted activity. In
the end of your presentation you talked about the "relief detector" technology, and I would like you to go a little bit further
in terms of some general comments. Whether as a matter of fact
technology is aided by an understanding of the way the human visual system or the animal visual system actually goes about
this? There are two aspects of biomedical engineering: one applied
if we want a physical system approach to problems and the other,
sometimes associated with science fiction yet scientifically almost upon us, the bionics approach, where we can look at the particular sensory system and ask the question what does it offer
in terms of new technology developments. So, if there are any general comments that you could make with regard to that point of the
"relief detector" technology, I will be glad to listen to them.

Mandar

I think that it is convenient to use a camera as relief detector,
because now the speed of the recognition is only about 10 lines
per minute and is limited by mechanical problems, especially by
the mobile head of the plotter.

Question (to François)

I would like to ask what are the perspectives for the market for
Braille production machines and what is needed in this market.

François

I will try to answer, but only for the kind of machines I was
talking about, not for individual printers. The machine I've shown
you is suitable for an organization, a library, etc. Considering
a country like Belgium, a Western country, a well developed country, we have in our country about ten thousand blind or partially
blind people, and the needs for those people can be covered with
about ten systems like the one I've talked about. That means for
one million people, you can certainly suffice with one system.
Now, if you consider this on a world scale, you have to figure out
how many people there are in the developed countries. We should
not export that kind of apparatuses to underdeveloped countries
because their infrastructure is insufficient. It will work for two

weeks, then it will stand there by lack of paper, lack of electricity or anything else. It will not be used properly. If we consider the Western world, then we have about 5 hundred million people which are potential users for such a system. That means you have 5 hundred systems in the whole world, and there are several manufacturers and each one of them will probably cover part of that potential market.

Silver (to François)

I'm sorry, could you expand on that? Do I understand that there are 10 thousand people who can read Braille in Belgium?

François

I don't think so! Ten thousand partially sighted or blind people doesn't mean ten thousand Braille reading people.

Silver

How many of them read in Braille?

François

I think about two thousand, at the most, and I don't expect that number to increase. Many people that are blind, are so because of old age, and they can't start reading Braille or it is very hard for them. So they rather rely on auditive systems and the like. I cannot give you exact figures on how many people restrict themselves to listening to books rather than reading books in Braille. I know the number of clients of Braille libraries, but that includes also people who listen to books rather than reading them by Braille.

Hertlein

I can give you some figures from Western Germany. We have a study from 1980. The survey found out that in Germany there are 75 thousand blind persons (in the legal definition of blindness); out of this number there are about ten thousand able to read Braille. But these are not the people who use it, only the individuals who read it. If you try to find out how many use Braille, you get an estimate of about 5 thousand. This is a very high reduction, and I think the focus of the total discussion is how many manufacturers we shall have to produce machines, like the machine in Belgium. We have Braillo from Norway. This is a very fast machine which is able to print both sides. We have the Thiel-machine in Germany and I heard that Triformation in the United States has developed an interpoint fast paper printer. The question is: how many manufacturers can survive in this market? That's, I think, the main question of this discussion. May I ask one question to Mr. Soede? You told us that there is a gap between man/machine communication in the computerized area. Do you know that there is a possibility to close this gap with a tactile read out? There is a German machine called MBT (Module Braille Terminal) that you can connect to any computer. With this device the blind are enabled to use nearly all the functions of the computer besides graphics.

Soede

I didn't know about this machine. I'm still wondering how blind persons can work at some factories. In fact, they have bought a tremendous amount of Apple, DEC systems, etc. How can blind people integrate in such factories and use the office automation systems as they are used in these factories? What has been presented now as a solution is probably not a solution in those situations.

Hertlein

I think it is, in fact, if it is the special working place of these blind men. They can do it with an interface connected to their personal computer and then they are able to communicate with the computer. That's possible.

Truquet

I should like to know the persons who are using compositor tapes, how they can use them. In France it's a real problem because the compositor tapes we have are not cleaned, and we have to clean them. Therefore, I think that there is a real chance for the optical readers, because even when they cannot recognize a character, they can make something on the screen to indicate the character which is not recognized. So, this could be a good solution to enter a document, because the compositor tapes cannot be used for all the documents. When you have footnotes and so on, when you have figures, it's a real problem. Only for novels it's interesting.

Werner

I am not aware of any case in which you have problems in reading compositor tapes. As to cleaning, the problem lies in the control characters inserted for formatting the printing. We had the advantage that these characters were taken out by the printing house in Hamburg before they sent the linotype tapes to us. It should be said that we got especially processed tapes because at that time the printing houses did not even have tapes which were supposed to be free of misprints. In fact, the misprints of inkprint were changed on line before they go to the press, without storing the corrected input. So, the errors are not removed from the tape, but only in the computer, when the layout is produced. What we've got were especially cleaned tapes. However, in Münster, we still did proof-reading and we found and removed additional errors. Nevertheless, I know that many of the errors in our translations are still due to the input.

Gill

The National Braille Press, one of the major printing houses,
just does 1/3 of its production directly from error free computer compatible compositor tapes. First of all, these tapes pass
through the preprocessor which is table-driven and the table is
set up for different printing codes. No printers use quite identical codes, but there is enough similarity to get away with
table-driven programs. The second stage is a program which goes
through and looks for errors. For instance, if you have a point,
you don't know whether it is a full stop at the end of a sentence or if it is a decimal point with no zeros after it.
Because in Braille, they are different. So, the program goes
through and every time it comes to something which is doubtful,
it puts it up on the screen and a human decides what it should
be. It does this for numerals, it looks for proper names, identifying capitals in the middle of a sentence and so on. This gets rid
of most of the errors before the text is translated into Braille.
If you want a perfect Braille, there is still no alternative to
the final proof-reading. The cost estimates are that it is 1/5
of the cost to do it from compositor tapes than to do it from
keyed input. For example, the National Geographic Magazine, which
we are producing in Braille has two unique problems. The first is
that the first character is missing from every article; this is
a huge character put in by hand in letter set in the final script,
so it is not in the computer tape. There is another slight problem that the computer tape has in a separate place the bit of
text which goes on the photograph, but this can be automatically
brought in. The second problem which is quite a problem is that
the publisher will not allow the Braille version, which is ready
two months ahead of the printed version, to be published before
the printed version. So, it stays on a shelf and when they phone
from New York that they are going to press tomorrow, the Braille
goes out that night.

Hertlein (to Mandar)

A very short question. Is it possible with your equipment to read
Braille from paper or from zinc plates?

Mandar

From paper and zinc plates.

Harres (to Mandar)

Do you have any experience with double-sided, interpoint Braille?

Mandar:

Only single face at this moment, but we are studying the case of double-sided, interpoint.

François

The system I've been talking about reads from paper, even if
the paper is warped a little, and even if it is not put down
straight. The computer takes it up in its memory and then starts
searching for lines and columns and rotates it until it gets the
maximum of Braille points, and then decodes it.

Truquet (to Hertlein)

You said that you have 80 thousand blind and so on, and you give
precise numbers, but in France it is not possible to have a precise number. We cannot know exactly the number of blind and the
number of low vision patients. By which process do you know exactly?

Hertlein

This was a study which was done for the Federal Ministry of Research and Technology (Bundesministerium für Forschung und
Technologie / BMFT) by an institute named "Infratest". This is run
by an organization in München and they found out these figures.
This study is available, if anyone is interested, from the Ministry in Bonn, in Germany. It is done by Mr. Hans Herzog.

Silver

Do you know what his methodology was?

Hertlein

No, I don't know exactly.

Werner

Let me just add one remark to the above figures. We are distributing the Zeit-Stern Magazine. It is a magazine for the blind,
free of charge to anybody who writes a post-card to the printing
house ordering it. The number of copies is about 5000. There seems
to be no way of increasing this number of actively reading blind
persons.

Truquet

I should also like that we speak in the next days of the maintenance of the Braille devices, of all devices for the blind, because it's a real problem. We cannot have a following maintenance.
We have a maintenance in Toulouse, because we have one of the
technicians who produce these devices, but in the other towns,
they have problems. I would like to ask Prof. François if he considered the problem of the maintenance of his device.

François

Of course, a machine which is both mechanical and electronic,

sooner or later wears out and needs maintenance, needs service.
Right now we have seven systems running, and in 1982 the average running time between interventions, between actions from outside, was about ten thousand copies. However, whenever something
happens, we draw conclusions from this, and if it appears to be
a child disease, we improve the design and we make sure that it
cannot happen again. We are fast approaching now a time between
maintenance, between service, of about one hundred hours. I think
it's a reasonable goal. That's one hundred thousand copies and
for most users this will be one month or may be three months of
use. I think it's quite fair if the technician comes around every
other three months, and takes care of the unit. In the future,
this will be organized on a commercial basis.

Truquet

What is the price of the maintenance and will it be annual or on
a call basis?

François

Of course, it is possible to do this on a yearly basis. Until now
we have done it on an "ad hoc" basis. If a system has a child
problem, then it is our problem and for the customer it is free.
If anyone has a normal problem, and in most cases it is transis-
tors or things like that, then we have charged a very simple cost,
most often no more than the displacement outside of Belgium.

THE ELEKUL BRAILLE SYSTEM

G. FRANCOIS

Kardinaal Mercierlaan 94, B-3030 Leuven-Heverlee, BELGIUM

ABSTRACT
    At the University of Leuven, a system has been designed
and built that produces Braille copies fast and economically.
The first two elements of the system, a text entry station and
a single-sided embossing machine have been operative in Belgium
since 1982. The design of two other elements is in progress: a
Braille to Braille copier and an editor for the automatic production of Braille.

INTRODUCTION : History of the project.
    The outset of our Braille project was a small flier,
distributed in 1976 by an organization for the blind in
Belgium. In this flier, a call was made for volunteers to
transcribe books and courses into Braille by means of a manual
embossing machine. Upon reading this request, we figured that
modern technology could make this task both easier and more
efficient. As a first step, we mechanised the embosser and
added an azerty keyboard and a cassette memory.
    We soon realised that this approach would never allow
satisfactory automation and we therefore decided to build our
own Braille printer. From the onset we took the option of
printing over the entire width of the page in one operating
cycle of the machine, thus producing a Braille reading line in
three machine cycles. This work got a good start in 1979, when
the Belgian Government, in an attempt to curb the rise of
unemployment, made jobs available for social projects. Within a
year, we put together a first prototype that printed one
reading line per second.
    We have used this machine to do some printing, however,
its main function has been to generate the guidelines for a
second-generation design with improved reliability and speed.
By the end of 1981 the last problems of this new prototype had
been solved. By then we had also switched from cassettes to
floppy discs for the registration of text and we were using a
standard microcomputer as an input station.
    In the course of 1982 and 83, seven systems were installed
in Belgium and in France, totalling 15 input stations. Experience with these systems has led to a number of improvements,
particularly in the software of the input station and the electronics of the embosser, bringing these two elements to their
state of maturity, which I will now describe.

The ELEKUL embossing machine
    The main features of the ELEKUL Braille printer are the
following:
    - High speed: 10 reading lines per second, single side.
    - The use of paper without folds or pin-feed.
    - High and uniform quality of the relief.
As in our first prototype, each reading line is formed in 3 machines cycles. The number of characters per line is maximum 40.
This gives a data flow of up to 400 characters/sec. The baud
rate for the communication with the source of information is

set accordinagly at 4800 bits/sec. Another way of specifying the production rate of the machine is the hourly output: more than 1000 pages size A4 or Quarto can be embossed in one hour of operation.

The limiting element in the speed of the machine is the stepwise motion of the paper in each machine cycle. During a line feed the acceleration and deceleration of the paper reach 10G. Both are quadratic functions of the speed. We have made successful tests at speeds up to 12 lines per second. This leaves us a safety margin of more than 40% in normal operation.

A second feature of the machine is the use of paper without folds or pin-feed. The paper is guided by a slot and moved by a roll covered with high-friction rubber. The elimination of pin-feed brings several advantages, the first of which is economic: paper on rolls is cheaper by a factor of 1.5 to 1.8. This is an important fact a unit that may use up to U.S. $10.000 worth of paper per year.

A second advantage is that the user is free to determine the length of the pages. The machine incorporates a fast guillotine-type cutter which operates at the command of the information source. Short notes need not use a lot of blank paper and for larger ones one page printed from edge to edge may contain, for instance, 1200 characters in 30 lines. This again means a saving of paper.

A third advantage is that after embossing, the bundles are ready for binding, requiring no further operations of cutting or tearing. This is an important saving of time and equipment. We also believe that rolls are easier to handle than heavy piles of folded paper, but the main point, in our view, is the saving of raw material: by omitting pin-feed and by cutting the right length that is needed, one will save on the average from 5 to 15% on paper.

The third important feature of the machine is the high and uniform quality of the relief. This is achieved by pressing the paper between a matrix and a row of needles with spherically shaped heads. The matrix is given a fixed displacement, independent of the resulting forces. The needles either move freely or are blocked by an interlock as shown in fig.1. As a result, the relief is virtually independent of the weight or the strength of the paper and we make it approach the limit of tearing of the paper fibers. Driving the matrix rather than the needles gives the advantage that moving parts are unloaded while parts under stress stay put. This principle, wich is valid for the interlocks as well for the needles, reduces the mechanical wear considerably.

The electronics of the embossing machine are grouped in a number of printed circuits according to their function. On the processor card we have a Motorola 6502 microprocessor, a 4Kbyte EPROM memory and 6Kbytes of RAM memory. Data is fetched in by an asynchronous communication chip via an RS 232-C connection.

The processor controls the operation of the machine, handles the data and monitors the front panel. The latter is kept very simple. After translation into Braille by the processor, the bits that determine the position of the interlocks and hence the printing of the needles, are sequentially sent to a power card.
They are stored on this card in latches and fed in parallel to the electromagnets that position the interlocks.

The magnets are mounted in two banks, one on each side of the printing block. The space available for each magnet is 6.1mm. The force of each for holding as well as for releasing the interlock and its spring is a factor of 10.

Power for the electronics comes from power supplies that are all of the switched-mode type. This saves energy and gives a cool operation.

The ELEKUL text entry station

The input to the machine is standard ASCII code, and it may be hooked up to any minicomputer equipped with an RS-232-C serial connection. However, none of the typhlophile organisations in Belgium had such equipment and they could not afford to buy it. Therefore we have developed the necessary software to compose pages using a low-cost personal computer.

The unit we have chosen is a TRS-80 from Radio-Shack.

Since there is a lot of excellent software available for more powerful computers, capable of producing higher-grade Braille, I will mention only briefly the characteristics of our entry station.

All 64 Braille combinations are accessible through the keyboard, which may be either azerty or qwerty type. The typist must enter what we call computer Braille, that is a character-to-character equivalent of the Braille symbols, and must apply the rules of Braille writing. He can enter higher-grade Braille if he wishes but still on the basis of an one-to-one correspondence, as he would using a Perkins or a Blista machine.

The program takes care of the page format, which can be chosen at any number of lines between 24 and 60. For lines of more than 32 characters the maximum length of the page is reduced to 30 lines. text is stored on 5 1/4" floppy discs, one diskette registers about 125.000 characters.

The same computer may be used for the input of text and for driving the embossing machine. In the latter mode the header and footer and the left margin on the Braille page may be chosen.

The Braille Copier

Quite often, the need arises to make a copy of a Braille text. Standard technology for this operation uses thermoplastics sheets and it only works for single-sided embossing.

The sheets are expensive and the touch of paper is generally preferred over plastic.

At the request of several users of our system, we are developing a copying unit that will read the original Braille text, decode it and send it out to the embosser for reproduction.

The original text is illuminated from the side so that each Braille point gives a well defined shadow.

The reading is done by a 600-line resolution television camera. The output of the vidicon is digitized in real time and stored in 32Kbyte of memory. Then comes the most difficult part: a microprocessor searches for strings of Braille points and attempts to maximise their lengths by performing a rotation of the page in its memory. Next, rows and columns are sought and, finally, the text can be decoded and reproduced. In fact it will first go to a standard input station where it can be registered, displayed and corrected, if necessary.

Tests on a prototype of this copier have shown that with

proper care, a distinction can be made between recto and verso points, so that we hope to copy two-sided embossing correctly bu the end of 1984.

The automatic editor

The application of computerized text processing to Braille production using files from editors or other sources may seem obvious at first. In practice, however, it is not a straightforward matter for several reasons.

First of all, Braille reading is very intolerant of misprints and the perfect word processor still has to be developed.

Second, the rules of Braille writing are complex and they differ from the rules for ink-printing, particularly when it comes to higher-grade Braille.

Third, the files of editors are most often coded by nonstandard formats, requiring special controllers and hence special hardware for each system.

Fourth, these files are seldom "clean", corrections having been made manually after phototypesetting.

Finally, the cost of the required apparatus, and the associated operating system is out of reach for many potential users and it certainly is in our country.

For all these reasons, we have abandoned our dreams of ever adding a fully automatic input station to our system. Instead, we are now working along another line.

The alternative to automatic editing is typing.

It takes an operator two or three weeks to manually transcribe a book. If we can somehow reduce this time by a factor of 3, using no more than a standard TRS-80 input station, we can break even in cost without any investment at all and in the meantime we can conserve employment. the operator takes care of the hyphenation and all but the most common Braille rules. He eliminates misprints and "cleans up" the file where needed.

The problem of special input hardware can be solved by physically connecting computers rather than decoding tapes or floppy discs. A one-day trip to an editor's office may give a harvest of 10 to 20 books.

We are presently working out the last details of this mode of operation.

Project Managememnt and Policies

All of the above is related to technical problems and specifications. We believe that the management of the project and the associated policies are at least as important for the user.

Our Braille project was started as a social project, intended to help the handicapped. Accordingly, we have managed it on a special basis, using publics funds and private gifts for the financing, and youth in civil service, students and unemployed for staff members.

The users of the system have paid only the marginal cost of manufacturing.

Our policy will be to follow this same path as long as we can, providing systems that are both cost efficient and of high quality. For the distribution and service outside Belgium, we have made an agreement with a local electronics company to work on an non- profit, break-even basis.

As long as we can manage it, our Braille project will remain a social project as a tribute to the memory of the genius who laid the foundations for it, 150 years ago: Louis Braille.

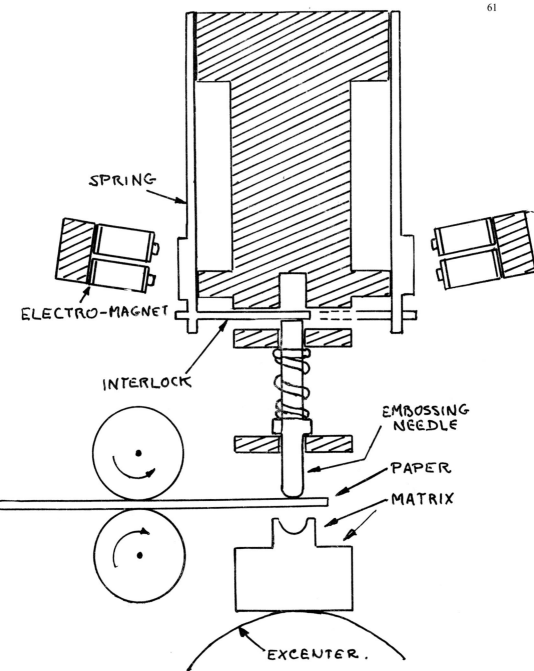

SPRING

ELECTRO-MAGNET

INTERLOCK

EMBOSSING
NEEDLE

PAPER

MATRIX

EXCENTER.

Fig 1. Sketch of the mechanism of
the Elekul Braille printer.

WRITTEN COMMUNICATION AIDS BETWEEN SIGHTED AND NON SIGHTED PERSONS

J.P. DUBUS, A. MANDAR, M. MORTREUX, F. WATTRELOT

Université des Sciences et Techniques de Lille
Laboratoire de Mesures Automatiques - Bâtiment P3, 3è étage

The present paper describes the design principles of some systems for the written communication between sighted and non-sighted persons. The systems presented are essentially the LOGIBRAILLE, the LECTOBRAILLE and a display with large size characters for the partially sighted.

I - THE LOGIBRAILLE SYSTEM (6)

It's composed of two parts: the editor-translator and the duplicator. The editor-translator allows the edition and the real time translation of ink-print texts into integral and abbreviated Braille. The duplicator is a Braille embosser controller.
The basic principles of this study were the optimisation of memory size (7) (4), the execution time of the software and the automatic transcription without any manual correction, in order to allow the use of the system by a normally sighted person, without previous knowledge of Braille.

The editor-translator principle

The diagram of figure 1 shows the principle of the editor-translator and the duplicator. Figure 2 offers the description of the whole system and its philosophy.

FIGURE 1

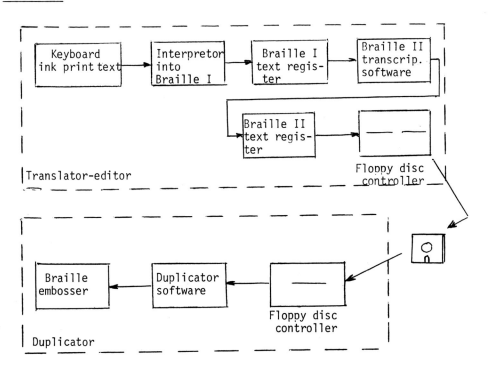

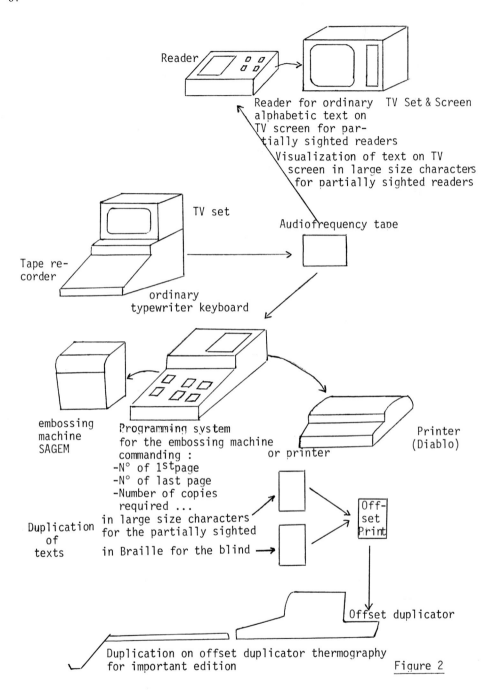

Reader

Reader for ordinary   TV Set & Screen
alphabetic text on
TV screen for par-
tially sighted readers

Visualization of text on TV
screen in large size characters
for partially sighted readers

TV set

Audiofrequency tape

Tape re-
corder

ordinary
typewriter keyboard

embossing   Programming system
machine   for the embossing machine
SAGEM   commanding :
             -N° of 1st page
             -N° of last page
             -Number of copies
               required ...
             in large size characters
Duplication for the partially sighted
   of
  texts   in Braille for the blind ⟶

or printer

Printer
(Diablo)

Off-
set
Print

Offset duplicator

Duplication on offset duplicator thermography
for important edition   Figure 2

Désignation	Syntaxe clavier	Visualisation	Braille intégral	Solution
Chiffres et nombres	4 382,5	4 382,5	⠼4'382,5	exécuté par logiciel
majuscules	Faire FAIRE ILE	Faire Faire île	⠘faire ⠘faire ⠘île	par logiciel avec de-mande d'informations
souligné nbre mots ≤ 3 nbre mots > 3	mots	mots	⠸mots ⠈mot ⠸plus de trois ⠸mots	touches spécifiques
n° 15 23°	n° 15 23°	n° 15 23°	n ⠤o ⠼15 ⠼23 o	par logiciel
1er 2ième	1er 2ième, 2ème	1er 2ième	⠼1 ⠤er ⠼2 ⠤me	par logiciel
dates	1.02.82 1-02-82	1.02.82 1-02-82	⠼1-⠼02-⠼82	par logiciel
ponctuations	mot ! mot! mot ; mot; mot ? mot? mot , mot, mot . mot.	mot ! mot ! mot ; mot ; mot ? mot ? mot, mot, mot. mot.	mot! mot! mot; mot; mot? mot? mot, mot, mot. mot.	par logiciel
A.V.H.	A.V.H.	A.V.H.	⠘A' ⠘V' ⠘H'	par logiciel
guillemets	"mots" " " " "	<<mots>> << << >> >>	<< << >> >>	traitement par logiciel et touche spécifique à fonction automatique
abréviations	M M. Mr Mr. Mme Mlle Melle Mlles Melles MM MM.	M M. Mr Mr. Mme Mlle Mlle Mlles Mlles MM MM.	Mr Mr Mr Mr Mme Mlle Mlle Mlles Mlles Mrs Mrs	traitement automatique par logiciel
tiret initial tiret final	—— ——	—— ——		
Caractères spéciaux	% ‰	% ‰		
Mots particuliers	Ils convient Il convient Expédient Ils expédient	Ils convient Il convient Expédient Ils expédient	(con)(v)(i)(ent) (con)(v)(ien)(t) (ex)(p)(é)(d)(ien)(t) (ex)(p)(é)(d)(i)(ent)	
1/2	1/2	1/2	⠼1 ⠌2	

Tableau I

The transcription of ink-print texts into abbreviated Braille is performed after its transcription into integral Braille. The abbreviated Braille is obtained from the integral Braille which containis enough information to be processed by the software transcription. The first job of the editor during the text edition is the performance of the compatibility between the ink-print and the Braille syntax. Table I is the résumé of syntax compatibility problems.

Both the ink-print and the Braille texts are recorded on a floppy disc.
The duplicator can drive a printer or a Braille embosser:
- the printer allows the utilisation of texts in large size characters for the partially sighted persons,
- the Braille embosser allows the utilization of embosser Braille texts for the blind.

The whole system has been commercialized in France and more than 17 organizations and schools for the blind are using it daily. It's used either for production of school books or reviews.

With the cooperation of the U.N.A.T. (Tunisian National Organization for the Blind), we have achieved the study and the realization of the same system for Arabic texts.

Nowadays most publishers have their book texts recorded on magnetic tapes. This tape can be read by a computer which takes from it only the text characters. In this case, the LOGIBRAILLE can be used as a peripheral for the translation (Fig. 3). The integral and abbreviated Braille text is recorded on a floppy disk which will be used by the duplicator to drive a Braille embosser or a printer. The printed Braille text is used to obtain a negative. In this case, the Braille relief is obtained by the heat of a special ink via an offset process.

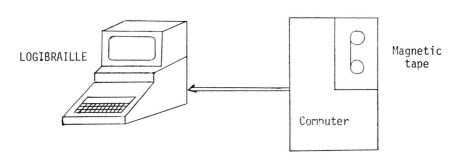

LOGIBRAILLE

Magnetic tape

Computer

Figure 3

This configuration of the LOGIBRAILLE is used at the CRDP (Centre Régional de Documentation Pédagogique de Lille, 3, rue Jean Bart - 59018 Lille Cedex).

In order to allow communication between blind and sighted persons, we have achieved the study and the realization of a system called the LECTOBRAILLE.

II <u>LECTOBRAILLE SYSTEM</u>

The LECTOBRAILLE allows the translation of embossed integral or abbreviated Braille texts into ordinary alphabetical French.

<u>LECTOBRAILLE principle (21) (19)</u>

A plotter is used as a support of the embossed text and its mobile head is used as the relief detector which is opto-electronical (Fig.4). This detector is composed of two elements.The element emits a pencil of rays through the lens L1. The second element is phototransistor sensitive to the rays coming through the lens L2.

When the reflection level contains the focus of the two lenses, the light flux on the phototransistor surface and the electric current generated are maximum.

<u>FIGURE 4</u>

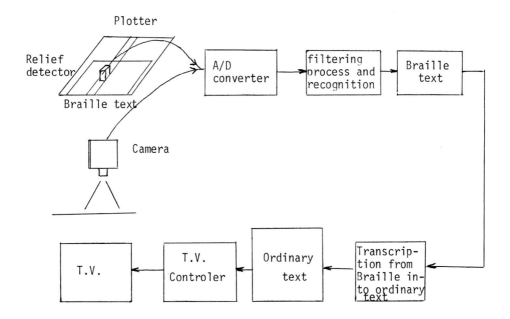

Figure 4

The curve of figure 5 shows the variation of the current generated by the phototransistor depending on the distance between the lens and the embossed surface.

Figure 6a shows the output voltage of an embossed sheet which is never perfectly flat. In order to eliminate this defect, we used a numeric filter and figure 6b shows the same signal at the output of this filter. This signal can now allow us to know if a Braille point is present or not.

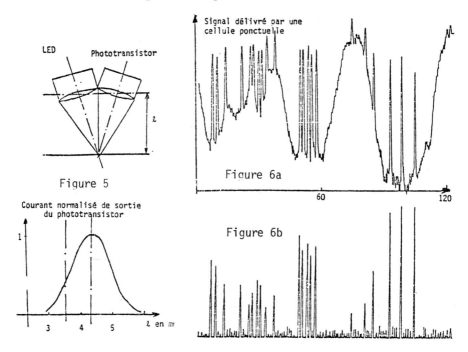

Figure 5

Figure 6a

Figure 6b

The reading speed of the system was increased by the use of three relief detectors.

After the recognition, the digital information related to the three detectors are used by software to achieve the translation of the integral or the abbreviated Braille text into ordinary alphabetical text. This text is displayed on a T.V. screen or printed on a printer.

The recognition and translation (from Braille to ordinary text) is about 2 seconds for a row of Braille characters and 60 seconds for a page of Braille.

III – VISUALISATION OF ALPHANUMERICAL TEXTS ON A TV. SCREEN FOR THE USE OF PARTIALLY SIGHTED PERSONS.

The objective of this project was the management of a T.V. screen in order to obtain alphanumerical characters of variable size being either seized from the keyboard, or a serial asynchronous transmission. The reader must be able to vary the size of characters, the space between them and the space between lines, in order to adapt the visualisation of the text on the screen with his personal visual (20) capabilities.

From a practical point of view, the maximum dimension of characters which is necessary for most partially sighted people is approximately 35mm in height or length. Besides defining a correct shape of characters, the minimum dimension should not be inferior to 7 lines on the T.V. screen, which imposes, for a 21 inch screen, a minimum in height or width of about 8mm.

We have chosen an architecture that should be able to satisfy these different needs, while allowing as low a price of manufacture as possible.

Figure 7 represents the synoptic description of the circuit of control on the screen. Such a circuit must manage the screen memory which contains the ASCII codes of all characters visualized on the screen.

That memory can, with the help of a switching of refresh address lines of the controller, or from the address lines of the microprocessor, in order to allow the writing of the text on the screen.

Figure 8 Shows some possible configurations of characters which can vary between 4 and 64 per line in a format which lay on all the screen size.

The texts to be visualized are entered either from a keyboard or from a floppy disc or magnetic tape.

FIGURE 7

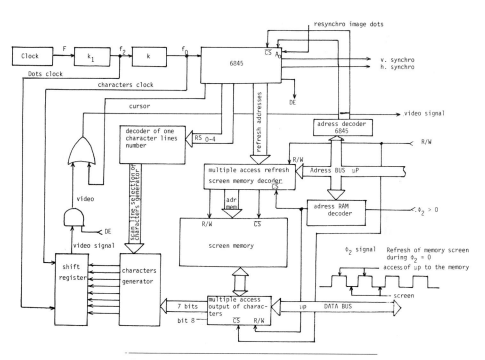

Synoptic of the architecture generating the videofrequency signal.

CONCLUSION

Two prototypes of LECTOBRAILLE are actually built in Lille. It completes the ring of written communication between sighted and non sighted persons. Seventeen LOGIBRAILLE systems are operational in France.

Recently, we built an Arabic version of LOGIBRAILLE operational in Tunis and we are working on a familiar microcomputer version at very low cost.

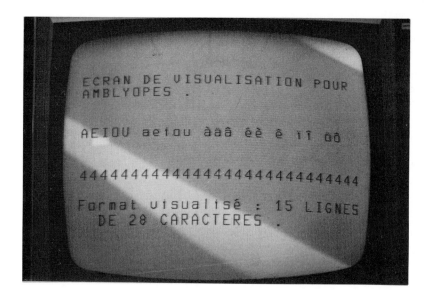

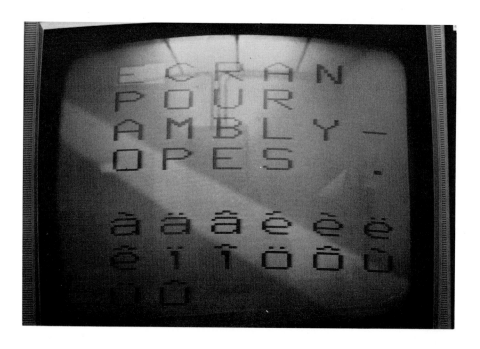

Figure 8

BIBLIOGRAPHIE

[1] BLANCHIN, HENRI, LEGUEVEL, Abrégé orthographique étendu. Ed. Valentin Hauy, Paris (1964), 38 p.

[2] DUBUS (J.P.), WATTRELOT (F.), Interpréteur-éditeur Braille automatique autonome avec clavier de machine à écrire, Le Nouvel Automatisme, Fr (Juin-Juil. 1979),pp. 31-35

[3] PAIR (C), GAUDEL (M.C.) Les structures de données et leur représentation en mémoire, 2è édition, INRIA, Fr. (1979)

[4] GOODRICH (G.L.), BENETT (R.R.), Computer access for the blind. Revues Tekniques - Tektronix (juin 1979)

[5] COLEMAN (P.W.F.), Tactile displays : their current state and a new approach. Conference international "on computerized Braille production today and to morrow". Londres (Juin 1979). Univ. Warwick, GB

[6] MANDAR (A.), Etude théorique et réalisation d'un système autonome interactif de transcription Braille. Thèse de Docteur-Ingénieur Lille, (22 avril 1982)

[7] DUBUS (J.P.), MANDAR (A.), Démarche adoptée pour établir la faisabilité d'un traducteur autonome temps réel Braille abrégé à l'aide d'un microprocesseur. Description détaillée d'une partie des solutions adoptées. Innov. Tech. Biol. Méd. Fr. (1980) 1, n° 2, pp. 4-20

[8] COURTIN (J.) Algorithme pour le traitement interactif des langues naturelles. Thèse d'Etat, Université Grenoble (1977)

[9] SNELDERS (J.A.H.), SPANJERSBERG (H.A.), An integrated Braille system Euromicro 1978. North-Holland, Amsterdam

[10] OSAMUN-SUEDA. Braille translation by micro-computer and a paper less Braille Dictionary. Conference internationale "on computerized Braille production today and to morrow". Londres (Juin 1979). Osaka Univ. Jap.

[11] BERTIL-MALBERG, Phonétique française. Hermods, Suède (1969)

[12] CARINALLI (C.) Slash CRT-Terminal component count with and I.C. controller. Electronic Design, 14 July 5, 1978, pp. 88-95

[13] DUBUS (J.P.),WATTRELOT (F.), MANDAR (A.). Description of a system for the edition and duplication of texts either in integral or abbreviated Braille for the blind, or in large size characters for the partially sighted. Sensory World, Lusby, Maryland (1980), pp. 11-16

[14] DUBUS (J.P.), MANDAR (A.), Méthode d'élaboration des algorithmes de traduction en Braille abrégé par dactylographie d'un texte. Optimisation de la taille mémoire et du temps de traduction pour implantation sur microprocesseur. Innov. Tech. Biol. Méd., Fr. (1980) 1, n° 4, pp. 53-71

[15] DUBUS (J.P.), WATTRELOT (F.), Etude de la visualisation de textes alphanumériques sur écran de télévision à format variable à usage des amblyopes. Innov. Tech. Biol. Méd., Fr.(1980), 1, n° 4, pp. 25-41

[16] CHRISTOPHERSEN (J.). The Nord Braille system. Colloque international
      Inf. et Braille (23-25 Sept., Toulouse 1981)

[17] DUBUS (J.P.), MORTREUX (M.), VINCKE (P.), SION (C.), Etude et réali-
      sation d'un lecteur optique de relief Braille avec transcription
      automatique en texte noir". Innov. Tech. Biol. Med. 4, n° 6,
      pp. 592-616 Fr (1983)

[18] DUBUS (J.P.), MORTREUX (M.), DURAND (M.). Méthode d'élaboration des
      algorithmes de transcription automatique Braille abrégé-noir en vue
      de leur implantation dans une architecture de transcripteur autonome
      Innov. Tech. Biol. Med. 3, n° 4, pp. 433-443, Fr (1982)

[19] VINCKE (Ph.), Réalisation d'un transcripteur automatique de relief
      Braille. Mémoire d'ingénieur CNAM soutenu le 26 novembre 1983 à Lille.

[20] DUBUS (J.P.), WATTRELOT (F.), A study of the visualization of alpha-
      numerical texts on a TV screen for the use of partially sighted per-
      sons. Microprocessing and Microprogramming 9 (1982), pp. 133-141

[21] DUBUS (J.P.), MANDAR (A.), MORTREUX (M.), Modélisation des règles de
      transcription Braille. Application à l'étude de processeurs de commu-
      nication individuelle entre voyant et aveugle. Annales des Télécom-
      munications, tome 38, n° 3-4, Mars-Avril 1983.

Différentes collaborations

Centre Régional de Documentation Pédagogique de Lille (CRDP) 3, rue Jean-
Bart - 59000 LILLE

Ecole Nationale des Déficients Visuels de Loos, Epi de Soil, rue Paul Doumer
59120 LOOS LEZ LILLE

C.T.B. INSERM de Lille, 13 à 17, rue Camille Guérin - 59000 LILLE

Association Valentin Haüy - 9, rue Duroc - 75007 PARIS

Session 2: AIDS FOR READING AND FOR THE INTERACTION

WITH CODED INFORMATION SOURCES

Chairman: H. Werner

"Ordibraille": A Braille Text Processing System
J.M. Lagarde, P. Lirou

Aids for Reading and for the Interaction with Coded
Information Sources
H. Doove

Applications of a Multi-Lingual Text-To-Speech System
R. Carlson, B. Granström

Multifont Textreading Machine for the Blind
J.A. Sørensen

Project for an Optical Character Recognizer for the Blind
A. Da Ronch, R. Spinabelli, A. Braggiotti

A Low Cost, Portable, Optical Character Reader for Blind
J. Conter, S. Alet, P. Puech, A. Bruel

Communication Aids
P.L. Emiliani

Design and Evaluation of Aids for Interaction with a
Computer Based Information Service
R.W. King

Discussion

"ORDIBRAILLE": A BRAILLE TEXT PROCESSING SYSTEM

J.M. LAGARDE, P. LIROU

"Langages et Systèmes Informatiques" Laboratory
University Paul Sabatier, TOULOUSE, FRANCE

INTRODUCTION

"ORDIBRAILLE" is a micro-computer mainly directed to reading and writing texts recorded on mini-floppy disks. It has a Braille keyboard and a Braille display. This portable and autonomous machine reduce enormously the bulkiness of Braille production and allows blind people access to computer composed documents.

Besides, this machine is a communication tool between blind and sighted persons owing to its facility for connection to a daisy wheel typewriter. It can also be used for communication with computers by means of its video terminal function. Moreover, "ORDIBRAILLE" offers supplementary functions such as:
- arithmetical computing,
- clock,
- automatic time switch, etc.

An experimental system is currently in use at the University Paul SABATIER in TOULOUSE.

GENERAL OVERVIEW

To clarify the following, it seems useful to remind readers that Braille encoding is based on three rows and two columns matrix of relief points: so 64 patterns are possible (blanks or spaces included).

These patterns set up Braille symbols. Sixty four symbols are not sufficient to describe the whole set of characters needed to write texts and formulae. So some of them, called keys, are used to modify the sense of symbols they are preceding (capital letters or digits for example).

In the past very clever electronic machines allowing reading and writing in Braille system have been perfected.

Paper embossing usually used in order to get relief points of Braille systems is replaced by a Braille display. The Braille symbols are recorded on cassettes in an enclosed form.

However, the chosen storing method leads to a lack of flexibility for updating and finding information. Indeed, in order to find a piece to be read, written or updated the worker must proceed the same way as if he were searching out parts on a conventional cassette tape.

Furthermore, modifications can be made without errors only if the number of Braille symbols to be substitued is equal to that of the replacing symbols (in the same way that it is difficult to exchange pieces of record on magnetic tape if their lengths are not equal).

These machines have also been built to drive a daisy wheel typewriter, an arithmetical computer or communicate with a computer, but for this purpose, it is necessary to add transcoding features.

The recent development of micro-computers helps to master these difficulties and to offer new ways of reducing the cost of this kind of machine. The possibilities increase through replacing cassettes by floppy disks and using current techniques of computer science and text processing. The price decrease is mainly obtained by the use of well-known components which are produced in large quantities.

The main function of "ORDIBRAILLE" is writing and reading in Braille. However, micro-computer support allows it to identify and to execute simple commands shared in four groups. The first group of commands deal with text composing aid characters:
- insertion,
- substitution,
- deletion.

The second group of commands allows the organization of the text on floppy disk by building a contents table. It simplifies information retrieval:
- beginning of a book, a chapter, or a paragraph,
- contents table listing,
- book-marker setting,
- book-marker retrieval.

The third group of commands intends making easier text printing on typewriter paper by providing the system with the necessary information:
- beginning of text to be printed,
- end of text to be printed,
- left and right margin,
- first line position of any page,
- number of lines to be written per page,
- justification.

The last group of commands give supplementary functions:
- clock setting,
- wake-up time setting,
- time gap to be measured setting,
- time display,
- arithmetical computing.

However, "ORDIBRAILLE" originality lays in the fact that all these possibilities are programmed. This conception allows extension of the functions of the system. It is also possible to employ it to fit the user's needs better. These facilities do not need fundamental modifications.

II DESCRIPTION AND FUNCTION
"ORDIBRAILLE" looks like a box the size of a portable typewriter. From the user's point of view, it is composed of a side aperture which allows floppy disk introduction, a keyboard, a Braille display, a loudspeaker and an on/off switch and connection plugs.

The keyboard is composed of the seven ordinary Braille typewriter keys (one for each point plus one for the blank), function keys are added to them for specifying certain commands:
- positioning on the following indented line,

- go back to the last line,
- back space,

for example.

The relief display is divided into twenty modules. Each module supports six movable electronically driven tips which represent a Braille symbol. At each extremity of the display lays a tactile key which displays the twenty preceding or following symbols.

The loudspeaker is used to give, by means of an audible signal, information about the execution of operations (end of delay, error,...).

When an error occurs, the audible signal is joined by a displaying message giving the error type. The connection plugs are used on one hand for connection to the electrical typewriter or to a computer, and on the other for taking its power from the mains.

When a floppy disk has been introduced into the side aperture the user can make "ORDIBRAILLE" run. At this moment, if a text is written on the floppy disk the first twenty symbols are displayed. From that time, the user can read, write or execute every command he wants.

When a Braille symbol is entered through the keyboard, it is sustituted to the one display on the rightmost module of the panel and the whole text is shifted by one position on the left.

The key "come back to the intended line" (respectively "intended line change") provokes displaying the beginning of the preceding (respectively following) intended line. if the desired indented line doesn't exist, the display remains empty.

Light touching with a finger on the left-hand side (respectively right-hand side) tactile key provokes displaying twenty preceding (respectively following) symbols. If there are no preceding or following symbols, the display remains empty.

In order to have permanent control of executed operations and to improve communications between blind and sighted persons and between computer and blind persons every character entered from the typewriter board or transmitted by computer may be reproduced simultaneously on the relief display of "ORDIBRAILLE". This facility is called "echoage", it is obtained by pressing the "echo" key. If echoage has not been required, the characters are stored on the floppy disk allowing the following operations reading, updating, printing on the typewrite paper, exchanging data which a computer or a French videotex system.

At all times, the user can ask for every command by pressing simultaneously the "command" key and a combination of Braille keyboard elements composing the letter representing the command identifier.

IV ASSOCIATED SOFTWARE

To drive all the machine components it was necessary to design specific kernel particularly fit to parallel processing management (for example reception of text produced by a computer and its storing on floppy disk with simultaneous display in the user's rhythm of reading).

Kernel functions are:
- processes management and synchronisation,
- interruption handling,

78

- memory managment,
- input/output management,
- application programs starting and control.

The system involves a file managment system.

However, in order to make the system modular structure apparent to the user and to facilitate the machine utilisation, a single module is affected to the interpretation of the several commands and to transmit them to the program concerned.

4.1 Text editing program

The editing program deals with collecting, storing and displaying the text with the execution of the operation on the text units.

It realises the following functions:
- collecting and storing the characters,

- text display management, shifting of one position to the display text on the left or on the right, displaying twenty preceding or following symbols, return to the preceding indented line, change to the following indented line,

- text processing operations:
  . insertion,
  . substitution,
  . erasing,

- contents management:
  . document recognition with a title,
  . chapter,
  . paragraph beginning,
  . retrieval of document chapter, paragraph beginning,

- document marker management:
  . position storing,
  . position retrieval.

4.2 Time management program

Time management program manages programmable clock and executes the following functions:
- time initialization,
- current time maintaining,
- time gap count (alarm, time switch),
- current time display.

4.3 Arithmetical computer program

Arithmetical computing program makes the machine be viewed as a scientific computer. Its functions are:
- conversion of digit string into numbers,

- operators recognizing and corresponding operation execution,

- eventually trace of calculation conservation on floppy disks,

- conversion of numbers into digits string result display,

- results display.

Arithmetical computing program is designed to treat most current operations. However, in order to increase its possibility, "ORDIBRAILLE" can be equipped with a computing processor in the form of an LSI circuit execution floating operations and numerous mathematical functions.
Several arithmetical computing program versions can be furnished in order to fit the user's needs: scientific, economic and statistical calculations.

4.4 Text formatting program
The text formatting program is conceived to automatically print texts on typewriter paper. Its functions are:
- suitable splitting lines and their eventual justification,
- titles and subtitles formatting,
- page, chapter and paragraph numbering,
- line printing according provided information commands.

This program was applicable to text reproduction on the relief display if the size of this one had to be reduced to twenty modules because of their high price.

V HARDWARE FEATURES
From a hardware point of view "ORDIBRAILLE" involves a 5" 1/4 floppy disk unit, a 15-key keyboard, a Braille display, a power supply, 3 cards nested in a mother board support the required circuits.

5.1 Central unit
The MPU board is composed by:
- MC6809 micro-processor unit and a MC6871 clock,
- 64 K RAM and 16 K ROM,
- programmable timer,
- two peripheral interface adaptors (PIA),
- two assynchronous communication interface adaptors (ACIA),
- WD1791 Disk controller.

5.2 Braille display control board
The Braille display control card supports the associated command circuits to the Braille display.

5.3 Keyboard card
The keyboard card supports the 15 keys of the keyboard and the "onshot" debounce circuitry.

VI CONCLUSION
"ORDIBRAILLE" has many applications in everyday life as well as in personal computing and in professionnal activities:
- books, newspapers, revues, dictionary reading,
- note taking (for courses or conferences for example),
- reports,theses or dissertation writing with word processing
- access to bank account statements, gas-meter reading, etc.,
- document exchange between blind and sighted persons,
- trigonometric calculation,
- clock alarm, time switch, etc.

This machine must offer new ways of employing the blind,
given the increasing computerisation in society (airplane
reservation or Videotex terminal utilisation for example).

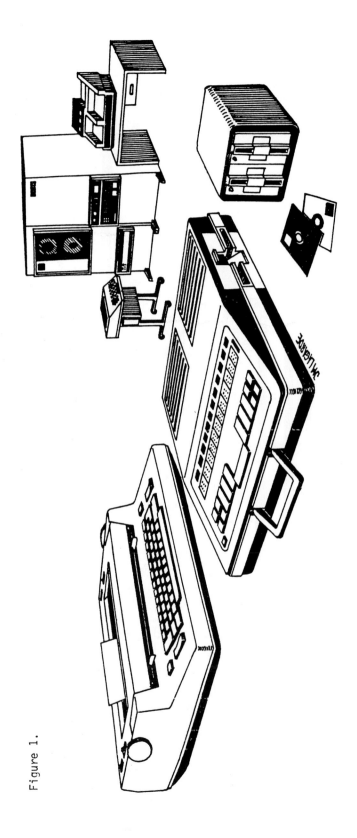

Figure 1.

82

Figure 2.

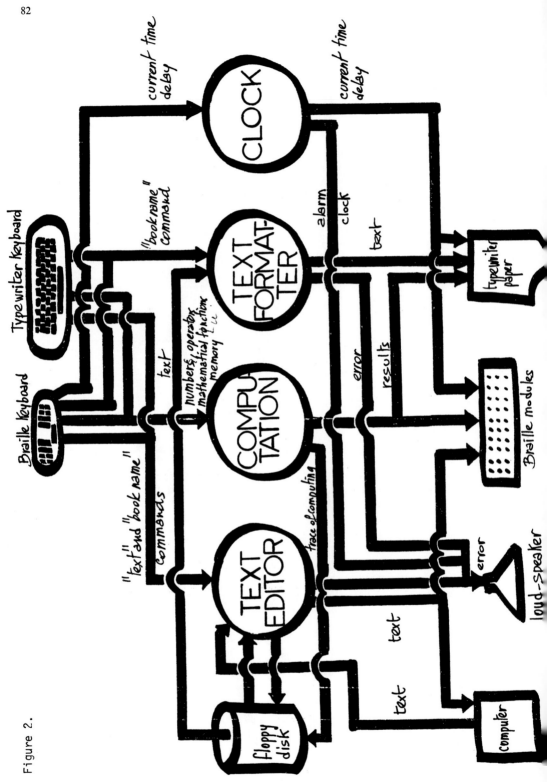

AIDS FOR READING AND FOR THE INTERACTION WITH CODED INFORMATION SOURCES

H. Doove
Netherlands Library for the Blind
Zichtenburglaan 260 - 2544 EB The Hague
The Netherlands

I would like to meet dr. Pier Luigi Emiliani's request to tell you something about the possibilities of braille reading, implying the use of coded information. Don't expect me to give a technological detailed treatise; I'd rather give you an overview of applications and devices, concerning which empirical facts are available at present; moreover, I'd like to cast a cautious glance at the future.

Unfortunately, it cannot be avoided that, considering the agenda, I will tell you things that you already heard, or that might come up for a more extensive discussion in one of the next sessions. I merely want to give you an overall impression of the devices such as are known at present, and as far as the Netherlands Library for the Blind, by which I am employed, has acquired experiences with them.

Since Louis Braille's invention in 1852, many institutions that are concerned with the production and distribution of braille as well as the individual braille readers have been confronted with the voluminous character of braille and its effects on storage. Solutions to this problem have been searched for. We know the "contracting" of different braille characters, grade 0-1-2; we know also the use of braille paper on two sides (interpoint); but in spite of these applications, braille books and magazins are still voluminous.

Today we find ourselves in the age of electronics, and, as for the production of braille, in the computer era.
In the neighbouring industrial countries electronics have been applied to information and documentation; now, the developments turn out to be useful to the production and distribution of reading matter for the blind as well.

Production of braille by means of a computer, where it is stored in coded form, means a gain of time, especially effective where reproduction is concerned.

At present there are several methods of converting black print texts, that is to say of translating them by means of a computer, into a coded form by which subsequently braille can be produced. The input to the computer takes place through a terminal, supplied with a keyboard on which the text is keyed. This terminal can be compared with an electric typewriter.
The input of the text can take place in two ways:

> formatted, that is to say, the text that should be put in meets lay-out instructions such as: the number of braille characters on a line, the number of lines on a page, and the right data concerning the abbreviation of words that can't be written in full anymore at the end of a line,

> unformatted, that is to say, the text can be put in at a stretch, whereas the lay-out instructions and word abbreviations are elaborated by the computer itself. The problems that occure here we have heard about in earlier sessions to day.

In case an input-terminal with visual or printer will be used, possible errors can be corrected before the text is written into the computer.

The devices the Netherlands Library for the Blind has at its disposal in order to put in, or reproduce the information stored in the computer are the following:

to punched tape:	an already out-of-date technique, by which braille characters are converted into a coded form. For the translations into braille a tape reader will then be required. The punched tape is a vulnerable medium, and rather slow in producing braille.
to magnetic tape:	offers proportionally much more storage space than the punched tape. Moreover, a magnetic tape operates faster, and can be used several times.
to magnetic disc:	can contain much more information, and can be operated much faster. To the finding of specific storages too, the magnetic disc gives much easier acces.
to a braille line-printer:	by this device the computer information is "retranslated" into braille, the line-printer printing braille characters with a speed $\pm$ 120 symbols per second. In Norway a braille line-printer has been developed, capable of printing on both sides of the braille paper simultaneously.

At the Netherlands Library for the blind, for the punching of synthetic plates a compact-cassette with coded information is used. It drives a composing machine (PUMA/EDV), that punches braille characters with a speed of 10 characters per second. The plate will then be turned upside down and punched anew (interpoint). After that, the wished number of braille copies will be produced on the printing-press.

Although these devices imply a fast way of processing, we are still overwhelmed by a huge amount of braille paper.
You might imagine what it means to the individual braille reader, if he or she would like to have, for instance, a braille dictionary, or even worse: a braille encyclopedia on the shelf.
On 1 square decimetre one can fit only $\pm$ 140 braille characters, whereas 1 square decimetre of a book's or magazine's text can contain $\pm$ 1.350 characters. The space problem is evident.

If I spoke just now about the coded form in which the text can be stored, it is exactly this form which offers the opportunity to put up a great amount of braille characters in a very restricted space. If this form of storage can be used for the individual braille reader, the space problem will thus be resolved for a great part too. It should be possible then, however, to make the coded information accessible again, that is to say that one should be able to read it again in braille.

A solution to this problem might be found in the development of paperless braille reading devices, some of which have been marketed at present. These devices operate with a compact-cassette (C60 or C90) as information carrier and this information can be read on a tactile reading line.

This line may consist of 20, 32 or 40 segments, each of them supplied with six movable pins that can form a braille character, and this generate a line of braille text. This requires high quality electronics, the tactile reading line itself is a mechanical part, of which all problems haven't yet been solved. The information on the compact-cassette has great density. Thus, by application of one C90 cassette 400 braille-pages can be stored. Moreover, these paperless braille reading devices imply the possibility of finding a page in the text, of getting up or down a page, in some cases of responding to a catchword, or of reproducing the text in black print through a special connection. These paperless braille reading devices are in most cases supplied with a braille keyboard, by means of which texts in coded form can also be put into the cassette by the consumer himself.

In 1983 the Netherlands Library for the Blind submitted some of these devices to a consumers' test. Generally speaking, the input of text, the correction of errors and the reading on the tactile line didn't meet with problems.

The presumption that these devices will have become common property before long, might be premature; for private use, the initial expenses are much to high. Meanwhile, these devices do find application as computer terminal, enabling the visually impaired programmer to store information from the computer in the cassette, and subsequently read it out through the tactile line.
The problem with these devices, however, is that the cassettes containing information can't be mutually exchanged on the various reading machines, because commercial backgrounds are involved.

For this purpose, a translation is required from one information code into another. In Sweden this possibility is already operational; in Holland a translating program will be started shortly. In cooperation with the consumers, the Netherlands Library for the Blind will put up a file of works in coded form on compact-cassettes. Dictionaries and other lexicographic works are the main concern.

Another development implying the use of the tactile reading line, is the transmission of viewdata. In Holland as well as in other European countries, we know two systems of transmitting information through television:

"Teletext", by which information in coded form is broadcasted along with the television signal, and can be made visible on a screen through a decoder built-in in the set.

"Viditel", by which information stored in a computer can be made visible on the T.V.-screen through the telephoneline and a separate modem.
Along the same way information can be sent to the computer through an inputterminal as well.

In both cases the information becoming visible on the T.V.-screen can be translated into braille. AEG/Telefunken in Germany has developed a terminal by means of which viewdata can be read out on a tactile reading line. This is of special interest for the group of deaf-blind.
AEG/Telefunken's device consists of a colour T.V.-receiver, a remote control and a terminal with braille reading line. Here again should be stated, that the initial expenses are very high.
On the initiative of the Netherlands Library for the Blind a prototype has been developed, by means of which Teletext-information can be read out in braille. This terminal, called "Braillotel", consists of a T.V. channel selector, a keyboard and a braille reading line of 40 characters, in accordance with the length of the lines the information is given on T.V. and supplied with 220V and an aerial connection.

At a later stage this terminal will be made suitable to "speech"-output too. The costs amount to about 1/3 of those of AEG/Telefunken's terminal.

To conclude with, I'd like to point out to a new development, which within some years might stand for a revolution in the field of talking books and braille books alike. It is the development in the field of the compact disc that's concerned here.

The Compact Disc (digital Audio) has a storage capacity of 600 Megabytes, which can be compared to 1000 floppy discs. On one compact disc 6 till 12 hours of spoken text (in coded form) can easily be stored.
The advantage of this system is made up by its world wide standardization. As a matter of course, its potential application as an aid for reading for visually impaired will have to be further investigated. The I.F.L.A. section of Libraries for the Blind will establish a working-group on this matter. It is encouraging to know that meanwhile negotiations have been started. The Netherlands Library for the Blind is one of the parties to the discussion.

Ladies and gentlemen, I hope I succeeded in outlining, however briefly, a picture of certain developments in the field of aids for reading, implying the use of coded information. Undoubtedly we are on the eve of as yet unknown technological developments. It is a good thing to keep eachother informed on these matters. This workshop offers us the opportunity to do so.

APPLICATIONS OF A MULTI-LINGUAL TEXT-TO-SPEECH SYSTEM FOR THE VISUALLY IMPAIRED

R. CARLSON and B. GRANSTRÖM

Department of Speech Communication and Music Acoustics
Royal Institute of Technology, S-1044 STOCKHOLM, SWEDEN

Text-to-speech systems have, during the last decade, attracted a considerable amount of research and development. Recently this work has resulted in relatively inexpensive products with decent speech quality. For the visually impaired, text-to-speech systems offer an interesting alternative to presenting text information as Braille or enlarged print. As production time and cost are essential, it way also be of interest for automatic production of recorded material. When increasingly more material will be available in computer form, the ordinary telephone could be used by the blind for accessing that text. Very little information is presently available on the use of these new devices. As a medium, speech is quite different from written information, whether it is in ordinary print or Braille.

In this paper we will describe the design and function of a multilingual text-to-speech system developed in our laboratory. We will also discuss some past, present and future applications of this kind of device for the visually impaired.

Different speech synthesis techniques

The application task determines the nature of the speech capability that must be provided in a speech synthesis system. When only a small number of utterances is required, and these do not have to be varied, some kind of coding technique is still preferable to true speech synthesis.

Speech synthesizers that essentially string speech sounds, "phonemes", together have been on the market for about ten years. The most well known manufacturer, Votrax, has recently managed to put a simplified version of their synthesizer on a single chip. Several companies are supplying chips for synthesis from a restricted sound inventory (allophones). These chips, controlled by a micro-processor with a text-to-phoneme program, offer potentially unrestricted text-to-speech capabilities at a very low cost. The quality of the speech has, however, limited the use of these low-end devices to special applications in games and, when lacking a viable alternative, in aids for the handucapped.

Research systmes with an ambition to synthesize speech in finer detail are now appearing as products. Speech Plus Inc. had developd a text-to-speech board based on earlier research at the Massachusetts Institute of Technology. Recently Digital Corporation has announced their DEC-talk also based on the MIT research. Both these device speak American English only. Infovox AB, a Swedish company in the speech technology field, is now marketing a multi-lingual text-to-speech module, SA-101; developed at our department in Stockholm (Carlson et al, 1982).

All these systems are based on 16-bit micro-processors and special signal processors for sound generation. The increased complexity pays off·in greatly improved speech quality that makes text-to-speech interesting in several new applications.

A Multi-Lingual Text-to-Speech System

Our ambition has been to comprehensively deal with the text-to-speech conversion process. We want to do this for any kind of text and for several different languages, in a way that makes the developed algorithms easy to implement in a portable system with state-of-the art technology.

Presently, synthesis systems exist for several languages: Swedish, English, Spanish, German, Italian, French, Finnish, Danish and Chinese. Some of the systems are still rather preliminary and imcomplete, while Swedish and English are the most developed. Many of the languages compare favourably with the speech from the best text-to-speech systemsm developed abroad. Even if there are obvious improvements to be made on most of the components in our system, the technique has come to a point where it is interesting to apply.

Different parts of the text-to-speech process have been written as separate rule packages that can be connected in an appropriate way by a supervising program. The basic configuration can be seen in fig.1.

User Lexicon

The input text is allowed to contain phonetic strings that are routed directly to the phonetic rules. These strings are delimited by special characters, chosen not to interfere with the ordinary text. After the phonetic text has been excluded, the input text is checked against a user lexicon. This lexicon can be changed by the individual user. In this way it is easy to add correct pronunciation to application specific abbreviations and other words that are pronounced incorrectly by the system, such as some names of foreign origin. The lexical entries can contain both ordinary text and phonetic spelling or a mixture of the two. The text found in the user lexicon is handled in the same way as input text, i.e., recursions in the lexicon are possible. This makes it easy to create very efficient individual abbreviation systems. The lexicon information is kept in CMOS RAM and is protected during power-down by a small battery.

Lexicon

The text then meets the "lexicon" which contains from a few hundred up to several thousand words dependent upon language. The main function of this component in the present system is to identify frequent words that usually are unstressed, the so-called function words. Exceptions to the pronunciation rules can of course be included and frequent content words can also be added for speed reasons. Strings that are found in the lexicon are changed accordingly and passed on to the "phonetic rules" component.

Number rules

In this component, digits and certain other non-letter characters are expanded to pronounceable phonetic representations and passed to the "phonetic component". An expression such as $4.50 will be pronounced as "four dollars

TEXT

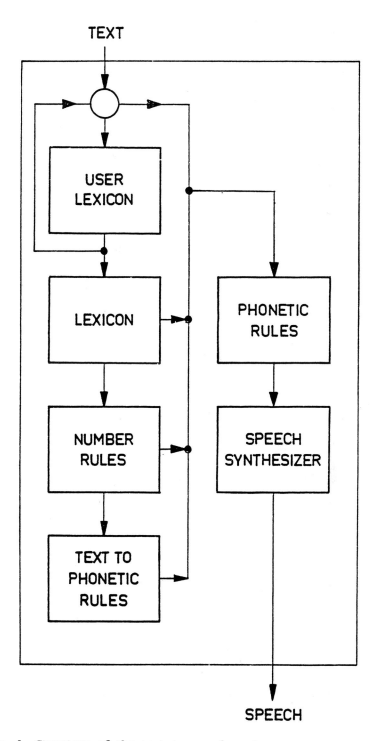

Fig. 1. Structure of the text-to-speech system.

and fifty cents". To some extent, this component is applica-tion-dependent. If, for example, a six-digit number is a telephone number, it should be pronounced differently from an amount and other rules are used.

Text to phonetic rules
This component processes the greatest part of a normal input text. The size of this rule sytem depends very much on the language. For Swedish and English, it amounts to several hundred rules. For Spanish and Finnish it suffices with about 50 rules due to the close relationship between spelling and pronunciation for these languages. This component operates on the "word" level, as do the earlier two. The output contains a full phonetic representation of the word, including information on syllable stress and accent.

Phonetic rules
At this stage in the process, the results of the three earlier components are merged and processed on a sentence basis. Phonetic realizations of the segments are adjusted dependent on context both within words and across word boundaries. Prosodic realizations including the fundamental frequency contour and the durational structure of the sentence are also calculated.

Speech synthesizer
Typically each 10 msec a frame of synthesis parameters is sent to the digital speech sythesizer. The synthesizer is a version of the OVE III synthesizer. It is a combined parallel/ cascaded filter structure with the possibility of mixed voiced/unvoiced excitation. A special feature is the dynamically variable "higher-pole correction", which makes it possible to model speech sounds produced with vocal tracts of different lengths.

Hardware realization
The present text-to-speech system consists of a formant speech synthesizer implemented on a signal processing chip (NEC-7720), a powerful microcomputer based on the MC68000 microprocessor and a variety of text input equipment. In the basic configuration, the speech module consists of four euro-cards. A stand-alone version of this system is produced by INFOVOX AB and is packaged in a 14X14X25cm box including loudspeaker and function controls and needs only be connected to a 5 volt power supply and any kind of text source such a conventional terminal or computer output. Two one-board versions are also available. One for integration into other equipment such a talking terminals or reading machines The other version plugs directly into the IBM personal computer and compatible machines.

Functions of the Text-to-Speech Device
The text-to-speech contains programms that make it easy to adapt to different applications. It operates in three basic modes: spelling, word by word, and sentence mode. Continuous reading at above 250 wpm (words per minute) is possible.
Besides the ordinary keyboard connection facility, there is the possibility of connection to a host computer. This is necessary in the talking terminal application, but is also useful in other contexts.

Keyboard commands to the system consist of a command prefix plus a command character. Some of the implemented commands are:
- Change reading mode: spell; word, line; sentence,
- change language: English, French, German, Italian, Spanish etc.,
- stop/continue output from synthesizer,
- change voice parameters: pitch level and dynamics; breathiness etc.,
- store/retrieve voices,
- change speech tempo,
- save/retrieve sentences,
- enter the user-lexicon editor,
- indexing of text,
- tone generation,
- inspect phonetic text.

Applications for the visually impaired

The generality of the text-to-speech system makes it possible to use different aids for the visually impaired. Some applications have already been tried but many more remain to be explored. To date (April 1984) some 50 SA-101 systems have been put to use by handicapped people. The Swedish Institute for the handicapped is presently running an extensive field evaluation, primarily in professional applications, and is planning on a report for late 1984.

There exist several possible ways for the visually impaired to access information through synthetic speech, some of these are schematically presented in fig.2. A centralized facility has the advantage of making the material cheaper to produce and uses standard distribution channels. Furthermore, the reader would not require any special equipment other than an ordinary cassette player. The only relatively large scale experiment reported in Sweden is an experiment with a centrally produced small-ad paper (Hampshire et al, 1982) which we will describe in some detail before turning to different applications.

Centrally produced synthetic speech

SRF Tal & Punkt, the production unit within the Swedish Federation of the Visually Handicapped, has, over several years, in cooperation with the Dept. of Speech Communication and Music Acoustics, carried out some tests with synthetic speech. The present experiment is part of a longer project entitled "Provision of Information to Visually Handicapped in School and Work". The purpose of this project is to highlight new information technology and its possible applications for the visually handicapped.

Previous speech intelligibility studies, with an earlier version of our text-to-speech system, have shown that the synthetic speech was readily understandable when listening to paragraph length material after some initial tuning in to the somewhat peculiar "dialect" (Carlson et al, 1976). Some subject reported a certain amount of fatigue after a long listening session.

Tal & Punkt is naturally interested to know more about the potential interest for centrally produced synthetic speech and the acceptability of the present synthetic speech for relatively passive listening.

92

In addition, more experience is needed of the actual technical production of such material, mainly in the editing of digitally encoded material to a form where it is appropriate to convert to synthetic speech.

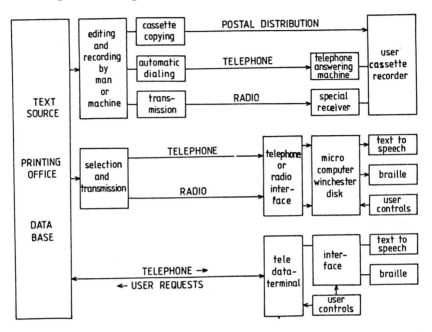

Fig.2. Different ways of accessing text by the visually impaired.

After considerable discussion and some preliminary tests with different kinds of material converted to synthetic speech, a weekly newspaper consisting entirely of "small-ads" was chosen for conversion and distribution in synthetic speech form over a period of four weeks. The main reasons for choosing this type of material were:
- the text was available in digital form,
- such material is otherwise not directly available at all to visually handicapped people (in Sweden there are furthermore, no broadcast advertisements),
- it is a material which is of potential interest to all members of the visually handicapped population, i.e., independent of age, sex, educational level, interests, etc.,
- the highly structured nature of the text. The paper was divided into about a dozen subject areas, each of which was further sub-divided into quite specific areas of interest,
- no realistic alternative method for making this material available to the visually handicapped existed,
- this type of text is difficult to read both for man and machine since it uses a lot of non-standard abbreviations, lack of punctuation and frequent spelling errors Our impression is that sighted persons are often in doubt of the intended interpretation of the advertisment

All subjects took part voluntarily. A condition for their participation in the experiment was that they should answer a questionnaire after the completion of the experiment. This questionnaire was conducted over the telephone and a 100% response was obtained. The age of the subjects ranged from 18 to 81, with a mean of 42 years. In total 75 persons participated (60 male and 15 female).

Results
Four issues of the paper were distributed. 95% of the requested synthetic speech editions reached their readers on the same morning as the ink-print edition became available. the final experimental edition included a total of 10 C-90 cassettes, which corresponded to approximately half the complete ink--print edition of the newspaper.

The time which subjects spent in listening to the recordings changed during the experiment. For the first edition 37% of the subjects listened one hour or more while that figure increased to 60% for the last edition. Several subjects reported that they actually bought things advertised, one acquired a second hand juke-box!

The reactions of nearly all the readers were positive, perhaps to a large extent due to the high motivation of the readers, which seems to be a very significant factor in acceptability.

The subjects' estimate of the speech quality is shown in Fig.3, where the scores are divided according to age. The youngest age group gives a somewhat higher rating of the speech quality. It is interesting that the post-retirement age group seems to understand and accept the synthetic speech fairly well especially considering the low penetration of Braille in this group.

Furthermore, what was particularly interesting from the point of view of the project was that there were many suggestions for what kind of material readers would like and would accept in synthetic speech, if this was the only method of making it available within the economical, practical and time constraints which existed. Examples of mentioned material are: continued distribution of "small-ads", encyclopaedia, telephone directories, zip-code listings, radio and TV programmes, time-tables for public transportation, recipe books, municipal information, mail order catalogues, etc.

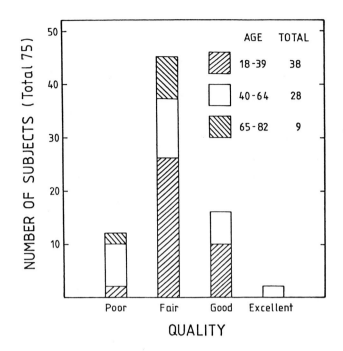

Fig.3. Estimated quality of the synthetic speech

Daily newspaper

Printing offices are currently using computers for type-setting most of their material. This means that the text is potentially available to blind persons after a text-to-speech conversion. One problem is that even a relatively small paper results in many cassettes. One ordinary newspaper will result in speech lasting for well over 24 hours. A pratical solution that is currently being implemented in Sweden is to make a strict selection that will result in only one cassette of speech. That material will be recorded by a human reader and distributed via FM-radio to special, but relatively inexpensive, equipment in the home of the visually impaired subscriber. This will, of course, result in a severe loss of information. The logical alternative is to distribute the text in digital form to the blind. That could be done on a telephone modem or as broadcasting, both making physical transportation of material unnecessary. The first alternative has already been tried and the second is now being implemented. The text is thus stored on a magnetic disk by the consumer. He could selectively search the material with the help of a small microcomputer. The text can be presented on either a Braille display or as synthetic speech. The personal equipment is today rather costly but it could be used also for reading arbitrary material. Library services could be extended to supply lliterature in digital form. With efficient search programs, this could certainly be an attractive alternative for sighted persons also.

Office work-stations

In cooperation with the Swedish Institute for the Handicapped and organisations for vocational rehabilitation several special work places for blind users have been developed. They are typically built around a personal computer, a text-to-speech system, a Braille display and printer. The goal is to gain experience on how such equipment should look and what facilities are needed. Very promising results have already been obtained in several office applications e.g. word processing, register handling and local switchboard operation.

Talking Braille recorders

The recent development of Braille recorders with editing and search capabilities has created a possibility for blind persons to interactively work with great volumes of text. Speech is in many cases a more convenient and faster mode of presentation than Braille. Giving this kind of equipment a speech output option has greatly enhanced its usefulness. It is today possible to package the text-to-speech device in a way that makes it possible to integrate it in a portable device.

Teledata and text-TV

The consequences of introducing (TV-) screen-based text information media have been discussed within the blind community. If the information would be presented only on the screen, that same information could be presented as Braille or synthetic speech, that could mean easy access to new data. As the teledata system expands, and efficient search facilities are implemented, it could be used as a means of distributing diverse information to the visually impaired, perhaps also newspaper material. One definite advantage compared to the systems previously mentioned is that no specialized distribution system is needed. The personal equipment will also be rather standard and inexpensive, consisting mainly of a small personal computer with a text-to-speech board.

A thesis project at our department has explored these possibilities. A small microcomputer-based interface box between the speech synthesizer and the Text-TV or teledata terminal has been built. A fundamental problem is the difference between the inherently parallel presentation of text on a screen and the consecutive presentation of information as speech. A special control box has been designed to make the search for information on the screen easy. The graphics that are not possible to convert to speech were expected to cause a lot of information loss. In practice, the pictures proved to be redundant in most situations.

Text-TV includes a facility to put subtitiles on ordinary TV-programs. This is important in a multilingual community and, of course, useful for deaf persons. Persons with low-vision and preschool children could, however, not use the subtitles unless they could be read aloud by a text-to-speech device. In many cases like this, when speech presentation is necessary for visually impaired, it could also be convenient for others.

Speech from bar-codes

Personal, cheap, portable and reliable OCR-devices are still far away but following the standardization of bar-codes, very inexpensive bar-code readers are now available. Some could be plugged directly into small personal computers. Many computer printers can also print bar-codes. This offers an opportunity also for the blind. Objects can thus be labelled and the information retrieved as synthetic speech. This is of course useful in some vocational situations but can be generalised. In shops mosts items are already labelled with bar-codes. The shop computer contains a register relating this code to a price and description of the article. Shoppers could borrow a portable bar-code to speech device with this information, when entering the shops. Just by scanning the bar-codes on different articles in the shop the person would be given the appropriate information by speech. This could greatly facilitate shopping for people with low vision. Work is presently under way to implement this facility.

Future of text-to-speech

As has been demonstrated, synthetic speech offers an attractive, alternative to enlarged print and Braille in many situations. Often speech should not be thought of as substituting existing media. It is rather a complement that will help in easing the information handicap of the visually impaired.

Today, high performance text-to-speech systems still lack some quality and are rather costly. The decrease in cost of electronic components and large scale production will cut the price drastically. Within a few years it will be feasible to include the text-to-speech capability in office computer terminals and other standard office equipment.

References

Carlson, R. and Granström, B. (1976) "A text-to-speech system based entirely on rules,"Conf. Record 1976 IEEE-ICASSP, Philadelphia, PA, USA.

Carlson, R., Granström, B. and Larsson, K. (1976): "Evaluation of a text-to-speech system as a reading machine for the blind", STL-QPSR 2-3/1976.

Carlson, R., Granström, B., and Hunnicutt, S. (1982): "A multi-language text-to-speech module", pp. 1604-1607 in Proc. ICASSP 82 (Paris), Vol. 3.

Hampshire, B., Rüdén, J., Carlson, R. and Granström, B.(1982): "Evaluation of centrally produced and distibuted synthetic speech", STL-QPSR 2-3/1982.

MULTIFONT TEXTREADING MACHINE FOR THE BLIND

J.A. Sørensen
Electronics Laboratory, Electronics Institute,
Technical University of Denmark, Bldg.344, 2800 Lyngby, Denmark

ABSTRACT

A functional description of a multifont text reading machine
for the blind is given. This machine is being developed. It consists of four main units; a page scanner with a resolution of
0.12 x 0.12 mm/pixel, a multiprocessor microcomputer system
which implements the picture processing and character recognition functions, a console through which the reading machine is
controlled by the reading person, and a Braille-display for
presentation of the text read.

The reading machine contains the following functions: Textline
search, variable pitch segmentation of the textline into isolated character pictures, 3 x 3 binary mask-filtering of unknown character pictures, size and position normalization of
unknown character pictures, extraction of geometrical features
of unknown character pictures, and finally a two-level classification of the unknown character. On the first level the features extracted partition a set of prototypes which is utilized
on level two in a nearest-neighbor classification using a modified, normalized Hamming distance. Furthermore a minicomputer
based character classifier design system which generates a classifier for the reading machine is described.

The reading machine is initially tested on typewritten text.

1. INTRODUCTION

The purpose of this multifont text reading machine is to facilitate blind persons' access to printed material - typewritten
or in print - by transforming this material into tactile information or synthetic speech. In the reference (6), J. Schürmann
gives a review of the reading machine area.

Fig. 1 shows the reading machine configuration to be presented
in the following. Here the recognized characters are presented
to the reading person via a Braille-display. The problems concerning the presentation of the text, when using synthetic
speech, is not treated in this paper.

From Fig. 1 is seen that the reading machine consists of a page
scanner, a microcomputer system, a console and a Braille-termi-
nal. The multifont character classifier parameters, covering a
set of typewritten or printed fonts, are transferred to the
reading machine via a minitape cassette.

This multifont character classifier is generated by using a minicomputer program system, shown in Fig. 2.

98

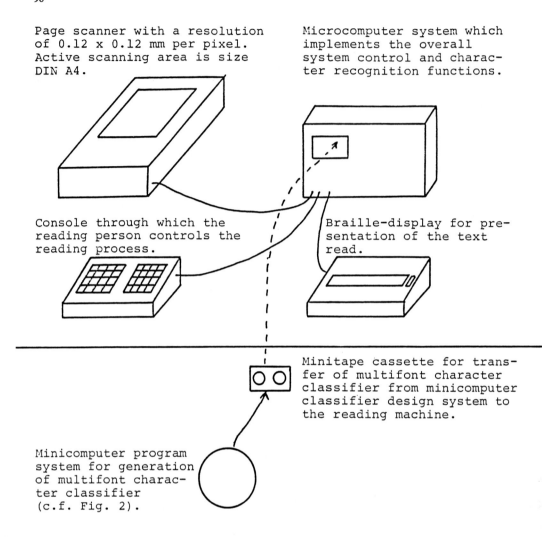

Page scanner with a resolution of 0.12 x 0.12 mm per pixel. Active scanning area is size DIN A4.

Microcomputer system which implements the overall system control and character recognition functions.

Console through which the reading person controls the reading process.

Braille-display for presentation of the text read.

Minitape cassette for transfer of multifont character classifier from minicomputer classifier design system to the reading machine.

Minicomputer program system for generation of multifont character classifier (c.f. Fig. 2).

Fig. 1   Reading machine configuration and character classifier generation.

2. MAIN DESIGN GUIDELINES OF THE READING MACHINE

In the following, some of the most important design guidelines for the multifont character classifier and the reading machine microcomputer system, which implements this classifier, are presented.

The character recognition method used must fulfill the following two conditions:

The character classifier must be designable using as input to the design algorithms a set of labeled characters, a design set, covering a set of fonts to be recognized. The amount of operator interaction during a multifont classifier design must be kept low.

Easy updating of the character classifier must be permitted during the reading machine utilization period, if a certain font is unknown to the classifier. This adaptive function is not implemented in the present classifier, but the recognition method used allows this function to be incorporated.

Furthermore:

The computer architecture used for implementation of the classifier must permit fairly easy enlarging of the available memory and processing capacity.

These demands result in the following two-level character classifier structure:

The classifier consists of a set of preprocessing functions performed on the unknown character picture followed by an extraction of a set of geometrical features. After that, these features are used for selecting a subset of prototypes among the total set of prototypes covering a multifont character set. These prototypes are transferred to the reading machine through the use of a minitape cassette. A nearest-neighbor classification is then performed between the prototypes in the subset and the unknown character picture using a modified, normalized Hamming distance.

The implementation of the picture processing and classification functions are performed on a microcomputer master-slave system of tightly coupled computers. Such a system fulfills the former demands for flexibility with respect to enlarging the available processing and memory capacity.

3. MINICOMPUTER PROGRAM SYSTEM FOR GENERATION OF A MULTIFONT
   CHARACTER CLASSIFIER

Fig. 2 shows a rough description of the minicomputer program system used for generation of a multifont character classifier. Furthermore, in Fig. 2 the sequence in which the programs are used during generation of a character classifier is shown. A page scanner, identical with the scanner used in the reading machine, is connected to the minicomputer. Using this scanner, a data set of binary raster pictures of characters is created by scanning books and typewritten documents.

For this purpose programs for automatic textline search and segmentation of textlines into isolated character pictures are used. These pictures are labeled by the operator and transferred to design and test files with binary raster pictures of isolated characters.

A multifont classifier is generated in the following way:
For each character class in every font a prototype is selected by determinating the design character in the class from which the sum of squared distances to all other design characters in that class is minimized.

Furthermore, a geometrical feature extraction on each design character from each font is performed. The features extracted are associated with the prototypes resulting in a two-level classifier, as already discussed. An efficient set of prototypes is selected so that the design set of isolated character pictures can be classified, using as few prototypes with associated features as possible.

Finally, the prototypes and the associated feature values are transferred to minitape cassette used for classifier transfer to the reading machine.

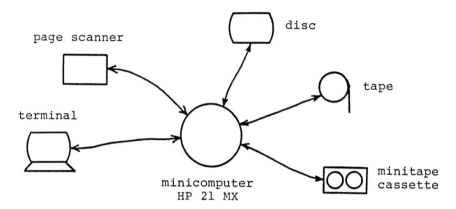

The program system for generation of a multifont character classifier contains the following functions used in the sequence hereafter:

1. Scan a page of text, search for textlines and transfer the binary raster pictures of textlines to disc files.

2. Segmentate textline into isolated characters and transfer these characters to disc files.

3. Operator supervised feature extraction on design characters.

4. Determination of prototype characters from a set of design characters.

5. Classify a test set of characters using a set of prototype characters and their associated feature values.

6. Transfer a multifont character classifier consisting of a set of prototypes and their associated feature values to minitape cassette.

Fig. 2   Minicomputer program system for generation of a multifont character classifier for printed text.

4. PICTURE PROCESSING AND CHARACTER RECOGNITION FUNCTIONS

Having placed a book or document on the page scanner, which outputs consecutive scanlines across the page in a resolution of
0.12 mm x 0.12 mm per pixel and 1728 pixels per scanline, the
following picture processing and character recognition are performed:

First the top, left and right edges of the page are detected.
Then a textline search is started and after having identified
the position of a textline on the page, the characters belonging to the line are isolated one by one from left to right
using a variable pitch textline segmentation algorithm.

The segmentation is followed by a set of preprocessing functions. The size normalization of the unknown, binary raster picture adapts the size of the unknown character picture to the
size of the prototype pictures transferred to the reading machine through the use of minitape cassette. Furthermore, the
unknown character picture is 3 x 3 binary mask filtered. The
purpose of this filtering is to remove salt-and-peper noise
from the binary raster picture.

Finally, in the preprocess the binary raster picture of the unknown character is position nomalized. The purpose of this step
is to reduce the computational load in level 2 of the final
classification to be described later.

The preprocess is followed by feature extraction implemented by
a state machine. The purpose of the feature extraction is to
extract rough geometrical information on the unknown character
picture.

The final classification is performed in two levels, where the
argument used in the first level is the feature values extracted
from the unknown character picture, and the argument used in
the second level is the preprocessed unknown character picture
itself.

In the first level of the classification, the feature values of
the unknown character picture are matched against a list of feature values associated with each prototype picture. If, for a
given prototype picture, a match is found, this prototype picture becomes a member of the set S of prototypes among which
the final classification in level two is performed. If, however,
no match is found between the unknown character feature value
and any feature belonging to the prototypes, all prototype pictures become member of the set S of prototypes.

Finally, in the second level a nearest-neighbor classification
is performed between the unknown character picture and all prototypes belonging to set S. In this classification a normalized,
modified Hamming distance is used.

Qualitatively, this two-level classification scheme has the following properties, assuming that the character font being read
is a member of the character classifier design set used.

Assume the printing quality of the unknown characters to be approximately equal to or better than the printing quality of the design set used. Then the mean number of prototypes per unknown character in set S, which remains to be exhaustively searched in the level two nearest-neighbor classification, becomes equal to the number of prototypes predicted from the design set.

Then assume that the printing quality of the unknown characters is poorer than the quality of the characters in the design set. In this case the mean number of prototypes per unknown character in set S becomes larger than in the former case. This decreases the classification speed, but still an acceptable classification error rate is expected to be retained within a certain printing quality range.

5. IMPLEMENTATION OF READING MACHINE FUNCTIONS

The two main units implementing the reading machine are a page scanner (1), (3) and a microcomputer system (4).

The video signal from the page scanner CCD sensor is binarized using a threshold which adapts to the reflected light intensity from the page background. The microcomputer system constructed for this application is based on a single master, three slaves, Intel 8086 multiprocessor system. In Fig. 3 a block diagram of the multiprocessor system is shown together with the main peripheral units. The address space lay-out of the system is shown in Fig. 4. Here the bus windows between the master computer and the slaves are represented by double or single ended arrows.

Finally, Fig. 5 shows the functional partitioning of the picture processing and character recognition functions among the processors. Further, the Petri-net in Fig. 5 shows the interprocessor synchronization of the computer system. The marking shown is the marking reached after system reset.

ACKNOWLEDGEMENTS

I wish to thank Professor Georg Bruun for many discussions and valuable support during the project period.

The project has been supported by The Danish Council for Scientific and Technical Research.

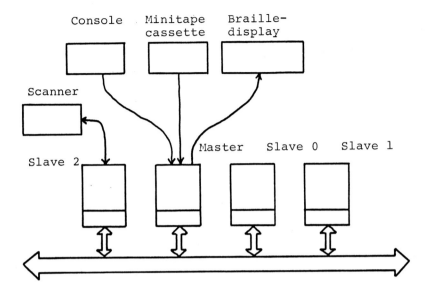

Fig. 3 Reading machine master-slave microcomputer system.

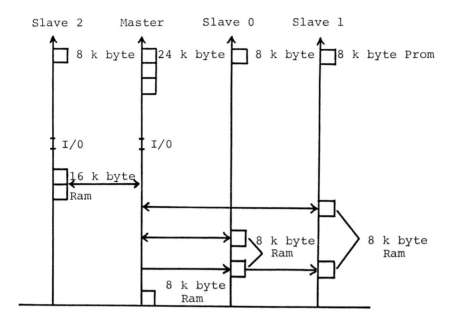

Slave 0 and 1 each have 8 k Ram addressable through two
address intervals for each slave.

The following symbols are used:

master → slave 0 → slave 1:
      write simultaneously from master to slave 0 and
      slave 1

master ↔ slave:
      read/write data between master and slave.

→ , ↔ : bus windows.

Fig. 4 Address space lay-out for the reading machine
      microcomputer system.

105

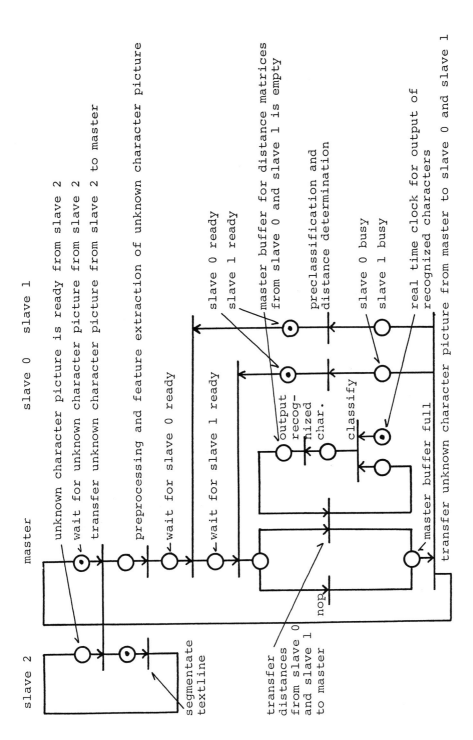

Fig. 5   Interprocessor synchronization for continuous
text reading.

106

REFERENCES

(1) Peder H. Krabbe: Inputsystem til læseapparat for blinde.
    Electronics Laboratory, The Technical University of
    Denmark, 1978.

(2) Vladimir Tchernov: Examination of the Layout of Text.
    Electronics Laboratory, The Technical University of
    Denmark, 1981.

(3) Peder H. Krabbe: Læseapparat for blinde - automatisk input-
    system. Electronics Laboratory, The Technical Univer-
    sity of Denmark, 1981.

(4) John Erik Aasted Sørensen: On the Automatic Recognition of
    Characters in a Reading Machine for the Blind.
    Electronics Laboratory, The Technical University of
    Denmark, 1982.

(5) John Erik Aasted Sørensen: Multifont Textreading Machine
    for the Blind.
    Proc. of the Third Scandinavian Conference on Image
    Analysis, July 12-14, 1983, Copenhagen, Denmark.

(6) J. Schürmann: Reading Machines.
    Proc. 6th International Conference on Pattern Recog-
    nition,
    October 19-20, 1982, Munich, Germany, pp. 1031-1044.

PROJECT FOR AN OPTICAL CHARACTER RECOGNIZER FOR THE BLIND

A. Da Ronch, R. Spinabelli, A. Braggiotti
Institute for Systems' Dynamics and Bioengineering (LADSEB)
National Research Council, Padova, Italy

ABSTRACT. A prototype of Optical Character Recognizer for personal use by the blind is described. It is based on microprocessor technology and performs multifont print recognition at a speed of about ten characters per second, with an error rate less than 5% .

INTRODUCTION.

The two most serious consequences of visual handicap regard individual motion and access to written material. For the second problem, Braille tactile code and voice recorded libraries do exist. The 'Optacon' is still the only wide-diffused device by which a blind may read by himself a black on white text, by means of a transduction from brightness to tactile perception of the images. In the seventies, the impact of microprocessors made it possible to think of digital computers for personal use as a realistic possibility, due to their reduced cost and size. An application of this technology was represented by the use of Optical Character Recognizers ('OCR') by blind persons.

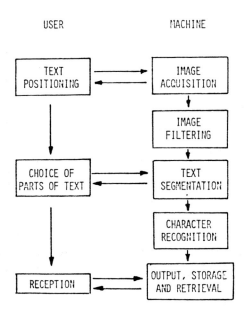

FIG.1:Man-machine interaction diagram.

108

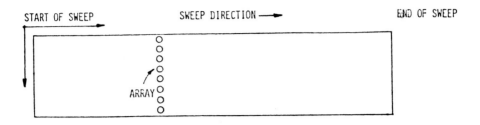

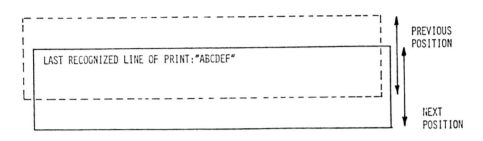

FIG.2:The action of the input terminal; the rectangles represent the strips of the text which may be accessed by single sweeps.

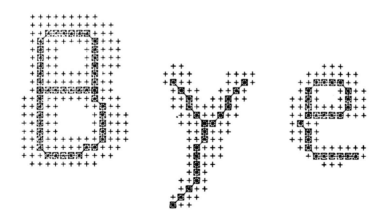

FIG.3:An example of thinning; crosses and squares represent the original images, while squares represent the thinned images or "skeletons".

At the Institute for Systems'Dynamics and Bioengineering of National Research Council, in Padua, Italy, a prototype of such an OCR is being projected. The operations involved in its use are summarized in the diagram of FIG 1. The device feeds the image of the text into its memory store through the input terminal and first controls if the orientation of written lines is consistent with internal X-Y reference axes for the subsequent operations; signals are sent to the user if correction is necessary. The so positioned and stored image is filtered and 'segmented' in distinct, uniform print areas (even a single one). The parameters issued from this operation remain available to the user for choosing the part to be actually recognized and displayed through the output terminal. Storage for off-line retrieval is possible too.

The functions performed by the device are described in the following.

THE INPUT TERMINAL.

The input terminal, which enters the information of the printed text into the processing system, is based on a moving head equipped with an array of 256 photodiodes, which scans the image through an X-Y motion (see FIG.2); this motion is controlled by the processing system itself, and allows the image to be scanned with a grid of 0.1 X 0.1 mm squares. The amplitude of the analog output signal is proportional to the average gray level in each element of the grid. This signal is quantized to a sequence of binary values obtained by comparison with an adaptive threshold.

Each sweep of the input terminal allows acquisition of a strip of text 25.6 mm wide and 204.8 mm long, and its subsequent conversion into a matrix of 256 X 2048 bits.

IMAGE THINNING.

The time sequence of digital signals generated by the input terminal is transmitted to a dedicated hardware device where the operation of "image thinning" is performed in real time (see example in FIG.3). This kind of filtering preserves form and connectivity of the sets of black dots on white background and allows for their description as graphs in the plane. The data obtained are fed into an input buffer in order to store the actual strip of printed text, for subsequent software processing.

SEGMENTATION OF THE TEXT.

The segmentation leads from the image of the text to the proper sequence of images of characters, to the purpose of recognizing characters one by one. It consists of three different steps.

In the first step, the image is examined to determine if it is divided into separate, distinct fields (headlines, columns of print, photographs and drawings). This operation is performed on an image of the text which has been reduced by a

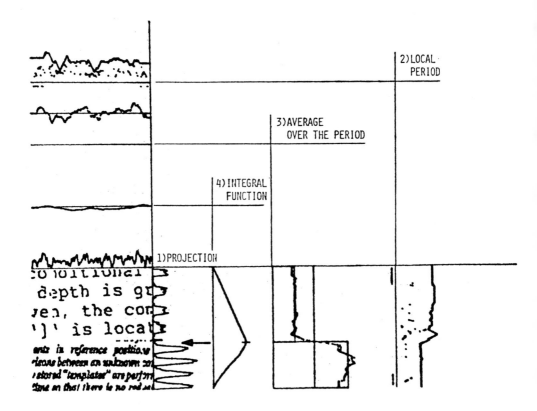

FIG.4:Detection of differences in print size. The algorithm is applied to X and Y projections (1) of square subsets of the image, and looks for significant changes in amplitude through such diagrams. To this purpose, each diagram is smoothed (3) by averaging over the local period (2); the diagram (4) is then obtained by integration of (3) and rotation until the last value reaches zero; significant changes in direction are taken and returned to the image subset as delimiters between regions of different print size (see arrows).

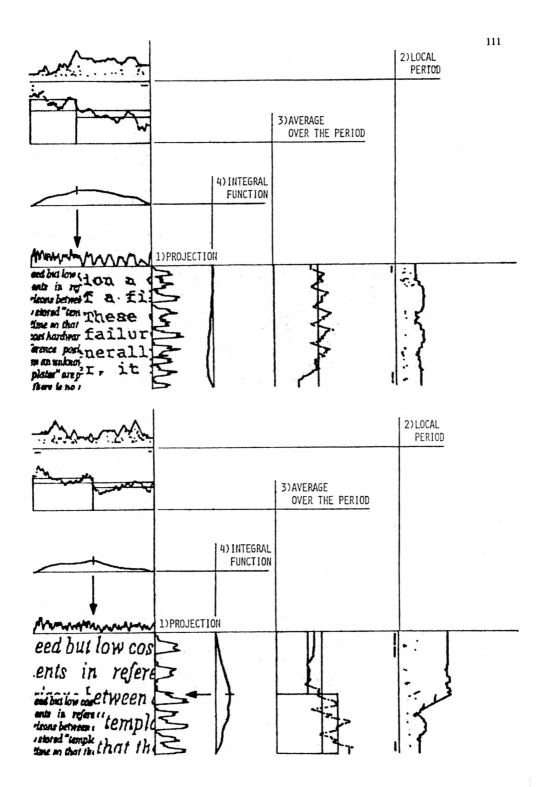

FIG.4: (Continued).

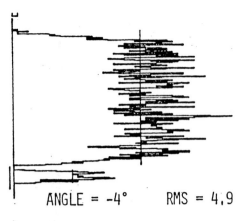

ROMA — Domani il presid
rà sindacati e Confindustr
niche per affrontare il co'
ima della scala mobile. No
nfindustria e sindacati siec
rte della Cgil c'è disponibi
adolini, ma non ad aprire
il lavoro.

ANGLE = -4°   RMS = 4,9

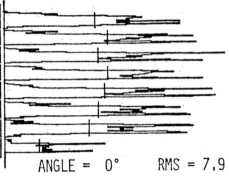

ROMA — Domani il presid
rà sindacati e Confindustr
niche per affrontare il co'
ima della scala mobile. No
nfindustria e sindacati siec
rte della Cgil c'è disponibi
adolini, ma non ad aprire
il lavoro.

ANGLE = 0°   RMS = 7,9

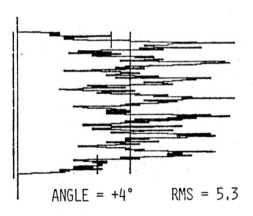

ROMA — Domani il presid
rà sindacati e Confindustr
niche per affrontare il co'
ima della scala mobile. No
nfindustria e sindacati siec
rte della Cgil c'è disponibi
adolini, ma non ad aprire
il lavoro.

ANGLE = +4°   RMS = 5,3

FIG.5:Segmentation of a strip of text (left) into lines
by projection on Y axis under different angles (right). The
RMS value of each resultant diagram is used as a measure of
black dots' alignement;   the angle corresponding to the
maximum value of this parameter is taken as the slope of
written lines in the machine X-Y reference system. Each
line is then considered as represented by a "single wave" in
the diagram; the result is represented by the segments next
to the vertical axis for Angle=0.

4 to 1 ratio, and consists of looking for graphic delimiters and relevant changes in the statistical properties throughout the image. As a result, major properties and coordinates of single fields are recognized, stored and made available to the user for the interactions involved in specific textual choice. The examples of FIG.4 refer to the detection of differences in print size; the basic assumption which is used is that, if the image is thinned, the black points' density increases with the reduction in print size. In the second step, the chosen part of the text is again accessed and stored in the form of subsequent full size-strips. The actual strip is examined to detect the slope and position of printed lines (see example in FIG.5). The slope is estimated by the evaluation of the maximum alignement of black dots; the position of each line is then indicated by a pair of parallel segments which enclose the line and have the predetermined slope. This set of parameters is used both to assist in the analysis of the next strip and to help in the third step, in which the single characters are extracted from lines. In such a step, each line is first considered as a sequence of distinct, connected sets of black dots; two different criteria are then applied in order to decide if a character is composed of more than one set or, conversely, if a set is formed by two or more characters.

CHARACTER RECOGNITION.

The thinned images of characters provide two main sets of features, to be used for recognition purposes:
1) images that have been normalized in size and position through a linear transformation in a 16 X 16 matrix (FIG.6).
2) topolgical data that allow classification of images as ordered graphs of oriented branches (FIG.7).
Each of the two sets of features is matched with the corresponding data that belong to the resident characters, for each of which a probability figure is evaluated; (see FIG.8 for mask matching); the two quantities are weighed and combined in a single score; the name of the best score's character is then issued as the name of the image being entered.
The resident characters' data were obtained off-line from labelled samples of characters by means of a set of interactive programs, consisting of three main parts:
1) simulation of the whole image processing;
2) cluster analysis applied to the population of samples (FIG.9);
3) estimation of the error rate, to help in the refinement of the functions involved in the two preceding parts, and in the evaluation of the number of samples which assured an error rate of less than the prefixed value of 5% .

THE OUTPUT TERMINAL.

The recognized characters may be displayed in sequence to the user, and stored on magnetic tape for subsequent use. There are two prospective methods of output: speech

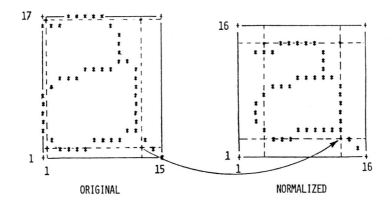

ORIGINAL   NORMALIZED

FIG.6:Normalisation of a character image. Each
horizontal and vertical broken line divides the original
image (left) in two parts, each of which contains a
predetermined fraction of the total number of black dots.
The linear transformation parameters are such to lead these
lines to fixed positions in the normalized plane (see arrow
left to right).

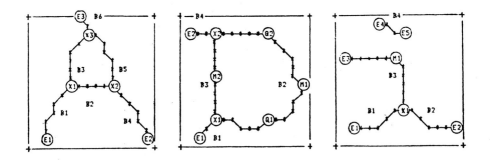

FIG.7:Topological description of characters. For
recognition purposes, each pattern is classified as a graph,
whose elements are: branches(B), crossing nodes(X), end
nodes(E). Some additional numeric data refer to the
normalized image: the positions of the nodes, the lenghts
of the branches; mid-and quarter points (M and Q) are used
only for long enough branches.

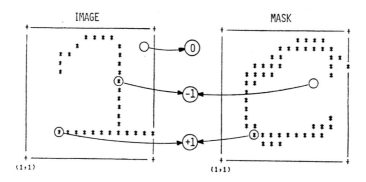

FIG.8:Image to mask matching. The score is first obtained as the sum of the contributions of all the 16 X 16 pairs of equi-position pixels; in the circles, the three possible values of such contributions are represented. A mask-dependent parameter, having the meaning of "expected score", is then subtracted.

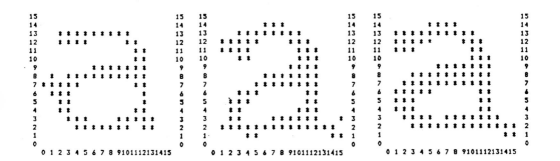

FIG.9:Some examples of masks as obtained by cluster analysis. A pseudo-distance is evalued for each pair of samples. A group of samples is taken as valid if no pseudo-distance exceeds a prefixed threshold. A dot of a mask is black when it is black in more than a certain amount of samples belonging to the corresponding group.

synthesis, performed by a dedicated processor, and Braille-coded tactile display, in volatile form,through a board of pin matrices. The output terminal allows for the above mentioned interactions, which assist the user in controlling the operations performed by the machine.

THE PROCESSING SYSTEM.

The basic requirements of the character recognizer, as outlined after a preliminary investigation,were:
1) the already quoted error rate, equal to or less than 5%;
2) a recognition speed of at least ten characters per second;
3) low cost and dimensions.
To fulfill the above conditions, the image recognition algorithms were first optimized for reducing execution time and memory occupation. To this purpose extensive work has been carried out on an ordinary minicomputer, using high level language.
The same programs were transferred later to a program development station based on an 8-bit microcomputer, and compiled in assembly language. A precise evaluation of time requirements was obtained this way. A prototype was then designed, based on a multiple processor structure of the pipe-line type, with one-way data flow, since the whole information processing can be carried out in an open-loop sequence of steps. This structure bears some advantages over the conventional multiple processors, in which a given number of CPU's share several common resources. It does not involve polling techniques, and can be easily divided into functional modules, allowing modular growth.

ACKNOWLEDGEMENTS. The authors thank Paolo Toffano for his expert technical assistance.
This research is being partially supported by the Special Project on Biomedical and Clinical Engineering of the National Research Council (CNR).

REFERENCES.

1) Yokoi S. et Al, 1973:"Topological properties in digitized binary pictures".Systems,computers,control.Vol.4,N.6,32-39.
2) Casey RG, 1970:"Moment normalization of handprinted charactes". IBM Journal Res. Develop. September, 548-557.
3) Da Ronch A, Spinabelli R, 1977:"Assottigiamento di immagini in tempo reale" .AEI Symposium. June,2/1-2/6.
4) Da Ronch A, Spinabelli R, Pagura C, 1981:"An optical character recognizer" .3rd Congr. on Medical Informatics Europe, Toulouse. March,876-882.
5) Braggiotti A, Pagura C, Spinabelli R, Valcher S, 1983: "Progetto di riconoscitore di testi a stampa per non-vedenti: il prototipo". Conv. su Ausili per Handicap di comunicazione, Firenze. March, 185-197.
6) Da Ronch A, Spinabelli R, 1983:"Progetto di riconoscitore di testi a stampa per non-vedenti: le procedure" .Conv. su Ausili per Handicap di comunicazione, Firenze.March, 199-209.

A LOW COST, PORTABLE, OPTICAL CHARACTER READER FOR THE BLIND
J. CONTER*, S. ALET, P. PUECH, A. BRUEL**

Equipe Vision par Calculateur du L.S.I.*** - E.N.S.E.E.I.H.T.
2 rue Camichel - 31071 - TOULOUSE CEDEX - FRANCE

ABSTRACT
This paper presents an optical reader for blind-people.
This device called D.E.L.T.A., ("Dispositif Electronique de Lecture de Texte pour Aveugles") is designed to enable the reading of any kind of font-type character printed for any support (plane or not). D.E.L.T.A. is the only operating system which is portable, and very easy to use. It does not need any training.
This optical character reader consists of a micro-camera with an internal tracking aid system. This micro-camera is connected to a specialized pattern recognition processor.
The recognized characters are generated in a BRAILLE tactile form, on a specific tactile output. The mean efficiency of the system is about 95% for most font-types. Reading can be operated at up to 15 characters a second, at the present time.
This system was designed with the constant advice of blind people.

KEY WORDS
CHARACTER RECOGNITION, BLIND, BRAILLE, OPTICAL CHARACTER READER, MICRO-CAMERA, MORSE.

INTRODUCTION
One area in computer vision which is especially useful to the visually handicapped is the detection and recognition of printed characters. During the past twenty years real progress has been made in the field of pattern recognition and image processing. Unfortunately, few systems for blind people's aid have been designed and commercialized.

One can distinguish three main kinds of systems.

1. Devices which are designed to store BRAILLE characters on magnetic-tape cartridges. These devices like DIGI-CASSETTE, BRAILLOCORD, VERSABRAILLE, can store a great amount of information, which can be easily retrieved, and reading of stored information is done by means of a BRAILLE display board. These devices enable manual storage of characters with keys and they are not designed to automatically recognize printed characters.

* J. CONTER & M. VALOBRA received the "Docteur-Ingénieur" degree for this work on November 4th, 1980.
** Scientist Responsable for this research.
*** L.S.I. is an associated Laboratory of C.N.R.S. (L.A. 347).

2. Another system called OPTACON generates patterns corresponding to the shape of the characters. The reader uses his fingers to detect the vibrating pattern of the rods activated by the system. This system needs a long training period for correct information reading.

3. The last category of system can be called "intelligent systems". Now, only one kind of optical character reader system for blind people is commercially available. This system is "KURZWEIL Machine". This machine can read any type of printed character, and its output is a synthetic English voice. The KURZWEIL Machine has been developed by KURZWEIL Computer products Inc., and is very efficient.
Unfortunately this reading machine is not yet cheap enough to be bought by the average blind person and, furthermore it is not an individual hand-carried device. To overcome the above problems we decided a, few years ago to realize D.E.L.T.A. which is an individual optical character reader, cheap, and able to identify most type-font characters, when these characters are separated by a blank column according to Fig.3.

I EQUIPMENT CONFIGURATION (Fig.1.)

D.E.L.T.A. consists of:
- a micro-camera with is tracking aid system and a preprocessing unit;
- a specific purpose processor provising automatic character recognition
- a BRAILLE tactile output to generate identified characters in an appropriate form for blind people.

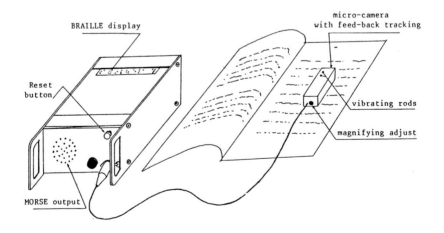

FINAL VERSION OF THE DEVICE
FIGURE I

1.1 The micro-camera and the preprocessing unit

First, we designed a special micro-camera for this application, using a 100 x 100 FAIRCHILD C.C.D. chip. In order to accelerate the information processing this"chip" was driven at a high speed (> 100 frames/second) and a specific hardware unit has been added to perform data preprocessing.

The visually handicapped operator is helped in tracking the printed line of the text by a couple of vibrating rods mounted on the micro-camera itself.

The vibrating rods are activated by the preprocessing unit:
- correct tracking: no vibration;
- deviation in the tracking: activation of the upper or the lower rod, according to the direction of the deviation;
- bad tracking, the micro-camera is too high or too low, the two rods vibrate (Fig.2).

FIGURE 2

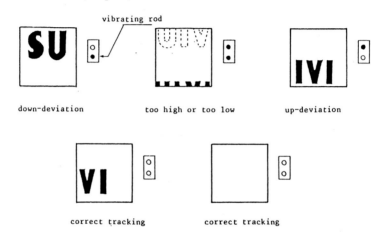

vibrating rod

down-deviation   too high or too low   up-deviation

correct tracking   correct tracking

TACTILE FEED BACK PRINCIPLE

The micro-camera is connected to the preprocessing unit by a flexible wire. The preprocessing unit provides three type of function:
a) Codification. The signal is real-time binarized. Pixels are grouped in words before being sent to the main memory of the processor, on a D.M.A. basis.
b) Synchronisation, transfer controls with the memory.
c) Frame analysis, frame selection, location of each character, extraction of some useful parameters. All these preprocessing functions are provided by hardware units.

These treatments are achieved in real time, with the sequential frame transfer process.

Concerning frame transfer we use two buffers:
- one buffer contains the last frame issued from the micro-camera;
- the other buffer contains the last enabled frame. When the last character seen by the micro-camera has been recognized, the buffer functions are exchanged.

The preprocessing unit has other important functions:
- it detects character separation;
- it gives information about exact micro-camera location on the current line by activating the two vibrating rods;
- it enables each character to be recognised only once;
- it can compute parameters such as pixels coordinate X, Y, character size, etc...

Figure 3 gives information on character enabling principle.

This data processing is performed at high speed by using knowledge of pixel locations in the photodedector matrix.

FIGURE 3

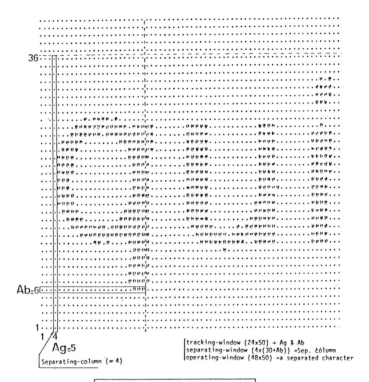

CHARACTER SEPARATION PRINCIPLE

N.B.

Unfortunately production of the 100 x 100 C.C.D. array has been abandoned by FAIRCHILD. So we had to design a new generation of micro-camera using a photosensitive array manufactured by THOMSON-C.S.F. (208 x 280 pixels).

Furthermore, to solve the very difficult problem of achieving the minimum size for this new camera we decided to develop an integrated circuit for the electronic command of this photosensitive circuit. This new component will be available in August 1984, and we hope, the future micro-camera will be assembled in September 1984. This important problem has considerably retarded the manufacturing of D.E.L.T.A.

1.2 Character recognition unit

It is not possible to find a perfect universal algorithm with a 100% efficiency. We tested a great number of known algorithms and because of their lack of efficiency for multifont character recognition we decided to adapt one of them with the following requirements:

-Efficiency 95% for any kind of font, except for SCRIPT or Italics. This efficiency is sufficient, due to the fact that the blind are able to recover the meaning of the sentence even with some erroneously identified characters.

- Reduced Computing time.
- Small size program, allowing microprocessor use.

our method refers to the methods using information extracted from the pixels issued by the intersection of the character with a set of straight lines. We used both horizontal lines and vertical lines for the analysis of the character to recognize; and in some ambigous cases we add metric properties.

FIGURE 4

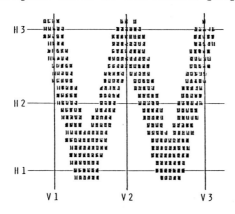

In addition, the resulting character codification is very simple, provided that position of the lines is well chosen.

We position the column in such a way that we can locate left, middle and right "down stroke". The only inconvenience of this method is its sensitivity to rotation and sometimes we can have trouble with an ambigous case for a non optimal location of the middle horizontal line.

In these cases we prefer to define several models of these letters corresponding to several signatures.

This algorithm is well suited to solving the recognition problem of characters with a serif such as TIMES, BASKERVILLE, SOUVENIR.

To overcome this problem the algorithm automatically detects this kind of character and replaces the previous column V by the new-one V (cf. Figure 5). Thus the character is assimilated to its pure form.

FIGURE 5

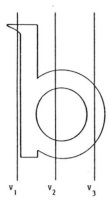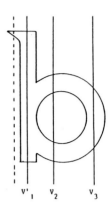

The pattern resulting from the intersection of each straight line with the characters never exhibits more than nine zones (black or white). A zone number greater than nine corresponds to a damaged character. In this case another processing module automatically restores this characters, provided the damage is not important.

II OUTPUT

Two types of output are used
- an audible output of the MORSE code of identified characters;
- a tactile output which is (temporarily) the BRAILLE display of the DIGICASSETTE. With this kind of display we can read simultaneously the last 12 characters which have been scanned by the micro-camera. This prototype uses a 6100 microprocessor and an all CMOS peripheral circuitry. These low consumption circuits are well-suited for a portable device with long autonomy time.

PICTURE 1 shows the present version of D.E.L.T.A. device.

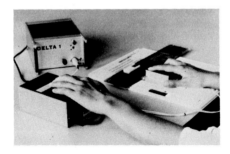

CONCLUSION

This system has been intensively tested by blind people. Now we are improving the character-recognition processor to achieve greater efficiency.

This system will be manufactured by the French firm SYSTELEC, so we hope it will be available on the market in the near future, despite the big delay imposed by designing the new generation of microcamera.

ALTERNATIVE SYSTEM: AN OPTICAL CHARACTER READER FOR AUTOMATIC BRAILLE PRODUCTION*

Efficiency and cost of BRAILLE production depends for a large part, on the ability to copy printed information.

This task is generally long and very expensive. Following laboratory experience in the field of optical character reading, we decided to design an interactive optical character reader. (seen in picture N°2). This experimental system is composed of:
- a linear microcamera constructed with a 256 pixels C.C.D. chip
- a low cost drawing table, supporting this new camera in place of the pen
- a MOTOROLA 68000 special purpose processor with an automatic pattern recognition programm
- a screen, which is used to display and control the generated text, identified by the system.

In using this kind of "feed back" on the screen we can guard against erroneously recognized characters. These erroneous characters appear in inverse video form so the cursor allows an easy, rapid correction to be made by the operator on screen before storing or editing the information.

Now, this experimental device is able to recognize 2 font-types with a mean efficiency of 99,5%. We are improving this system by using a special module which can automatically generate a new dictionary of "signatures", allowing reading of new font-type characters.

Our main goal was to design an interactive system at a very low price, compared with the optical character readers now commercially available.

This table reports the first results in testing this optical character reader.

Font	Type	Intercharacter distance	Efficiency
IBM Letter Gothic	Original	12 cps	99,6 or 99,1%
IBM Letter Gothic	Photocopy	12 cps	98,9%
IBM Prestige Elite	Original	12 cps	97,1%
IBM Prestige Elite	Photocopy	10 cps	98,5%

We are improving the efficiency of this reader, and we think it will be manufactured in the near future by ELAN INFORMATIQUE FIRM, which has been cooperating on this project for a few months.

CONLCUSION

This last device could be very useful in a Braille Production Station. At the moment we are improving these systems in collaboration with industrial partners. The automatic pattern recognition part of the system has some very difficult problems still to be solved, so we will have to spend a lot of time to achieve a perfect system which will be able to make a faultless interpretation.

* For this work Mr. VICTORIA, received the "Docteur de 3° Cycle" on November 24th, 1983.

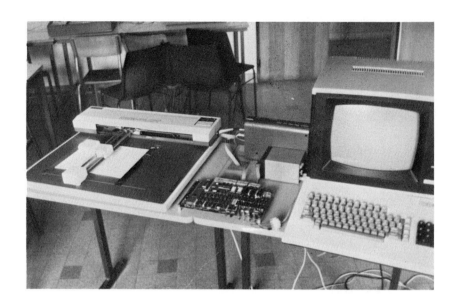

Picture 2

BIBLIOGRAPHIE

S. CASTAN et G. PERENNOU
Reconnaissance structurelle de graphisme
Congrès AFCET-IRIA (1978)

A. CHEHIKIAN
Un procédé de reconnaissance structurelle des caractères alphanumériques.
Congrès AFCET-IRIA (1978)

J. CONTER, M. VALOBRA
D.E.L.T.A. : Dispositif Electronique de Lecture de Textes pour Aveugles.
Système portatif multifonte. Thèse de Docteur-Ingénieur. I.N.P.-U.P.S.
TOULOUSE. 1980.

H. FREEMAN
On the encodinf of arbitrary geometric configurations.
I.E.E.E. Transactions Electronics Computer. 1961.

H. FREIBERGER
Research Protheses and Sensory aids for the Blind.
"8th annual Automatic Image Pattern Recognition Symposium Proceedings"
3-4 Avril 1978.

K.S. FU
Syntactic Methods in Pattern Recognition. Academic Press (1974).

G. GAILLAT-M. BERTHOD
Panorama des techniques d'extraction de traits caractéristiques en lecture
optique.
Congrès AFCET-IRIA 1979.

K. ISHII, K. KANEMAKI, K. KOMORI (Nippon Telegraph Yokosuka Japon)
Automatic Design of a Character Recognition Dictionnary Based on Feature
Concentration Method. 4 th. IJCPR. TOKYO 1978.

KURZWEIL COMPUTER PRODUCTS. Cambridge. Massachussetts.
Science Writers Seminar in Ophtalmology. 8-11 Mai 1976.

LOPEZ-KRAHE
Etude expérimentale d'une méthode de reconnaissance. 1° Congrès AFCET-IRIA.
PARIS 1978.

LOPEZ-KRAHE
Etude de méthodes de reconnaissance automatique de caractères imprimés. Application à un système de lecture pour aveugles. Thèse présentée à l'Université de PARIS VIII en avril 1979.

Ph. MARTHON, A. BRUEL, G. BIGUET
Squelettisation par calcul d'une fonction discriminante sur un voisinage de
huit points. Congrès AFCET-IRIA. TOULOUSE. Septembre 1979.

J.H. MUMSON, R.E. SAVOIE, R.P. SHEPARD
System study of an interactive computer. Aided, text reading service for the
blind available through any telephone.
National Institutes of the Health. Stanford Research Institute.

POSTE TELEGRAPHE, TELEPHONE DES PAYS BAS
Méthode pour la reconnaissance de caractères.

M. RAHIER, P.G.A. JESPERS
Microelectronics Laboratories. Catholic University of Louvain. Belgium.
A low cost hand-carried OCR system implemented with monolithic IC's
4 th IJCPR. TOKYO 1978.

J.C. SIMON
A short survey of character recognition NATO advanced study institute on
digital image processing. BONAS 1976.

SCHNEIDER-MAUNOURY. Secrétaire Général de l'Association Valentin HAUY.
Rapport sur l'écriture Braille à l'âge électronique : digicassettes, calcu-
latrices et production de Braille par ordinateur (Novembre 1978).

B. THIESSE, Ph. MARTHON, A. BRUEL
Recherche optimale de points caractéristiques dans un dictionnaire d'images.
Congrès AFCET-IRIA. 12-14 Septembre 1979. TOULOUSE.

T. VO VAN
Une méthode de reconnaissance de caractères (latins et chinois) non stylisés.
Congrès AFCET-IRIA. 1978.

J. CONTER, M. VALOBRA, A. BRUEL
A low cost, portable, optical character reader for blind. Conference on pattern recognition and image processing. August 1981. DALLAS. U.S.A.

A. BRUEL, J. CONTER, M. VALOBRA
Procédé de lecture pour non-voyants et dispositif pour la mise en oeuvre du
procédé. Brevet d'invention n° 80.23771. 4 Novembre 1980.

G. VICTORIA
Saisie interactive de textes par lecture optique de caractères. Application
à la réalisation d'une maquette probatoire de lecteur pour la bureautique.
Thèse de 3° Cycle. Université Paul Sabatier. Toulouse. Novembre 1983.

COMMUNICATION AIDS

P.L. Emiliani
Istituto di Ricerca sulle Onde Elettromagnetiche (I.R.O.E.)
Consiglio Nazionale delle Ricerche (C.N.R.)
Via Panciatichi 64, 50127 Firenze, Italy

1) Introduction

The Italian research and development activity in the field
of communication aids for the blind is reviewed, mainly considering the work in the Special Projects on Biomedical Engineering,
research structures which have been active in Italy for several
years.

The results obtained in the development of technical aids, in
the elaboration of training techniques, in setting up procedures
for the evaluation of aids and of the resulting rehabilitation
levels, and in working out different rehabilitation methodologies
are considered.

Some considerations about the problem of the development of
aids which are based on microprocessors and use signal processing
techniques (e.g. speech processing) are presented, examining
their design, use and relevance in the access to education and
culture and in vocational training.

2) Research and development in communication aids for the blind
   in the Special Projects on Biomedical Engineering

The Special Projects of the Italian National Research Council
(CNR) were started in 1976, in order to set up coordinated programs in applied research, with the cooperation of research groups
at the CNR, Universities and other organizations, and of industrial groups in companies active in this sector. The main purpose was
to create a link between research and production and, therefore,
to have a transfer of innovative ideas from research to production
and an input of important practical issues in the reverse direction.

Among the selected sectors, a Special Project was started in
Biomedical Engineering, under the direction of Prof. L. Donato.
One of its subprojects was devoted to the research and development in communication aids and, under the coordination of Prof.
G. Gambardella, some interesting results were obtained which are
described in the following. In a second and more recent Special
Project on Biomedical and Clinical Engineering, started in 1983,
a new subproject on communication aids was included, under the coordination of the author, whose activities we are also reviewing.

a) Speech synthesis applications

This research program was started in 1978 within the previously mentioned Special Project and a prototype of a text-to-speech system for the Italian language was built at the IROE, to be used for the interaction of the blind with a source of coded information (computer, data bank, etc.), thus increasing their possibilities in the access to education, culture and work [1].

The implemented hardware uses an approach to voice synthesis, which was developed several years ago at the Padua University to obtain a monotonous but highly intelligible synthetic speech and is based on the concatenation of Standard Speech Reproducing Units (SSRUs) for the Italian language [2], coded using the LPC technique [3]. The system is based on a Z80 microprocessor for the acquisition of characters, the conversion from normal to phonetic alphabet and the singling out of the SSRUs, and on a bit-slice arithmetic structure to implement the synthesis lattice filter.

The prototype has been acquired by an Italian company (TXT Software & Telematica - Milano), which recently started a normal industrial production.

At present, the activity at the IROE in this field is mainly devoted to the development of the interaction software and to its testing in different real applications (computer programming, access to data banks), while at the Electronics Engineering Department of the University in Padua studies are devoted to the problem of the introduction of prosody in the synthesized language and the production of better sets of SSRUs. New hardware structures are also studied to obtain simpler and less expensive synthesizers.

b) Reading machine for the blind

A prototype of a reading machine for the blind is under development at the Institute for the Research on the Dynamics of Systems and Bioengineering of the CNR in Padua, where the scanner for the automatic acquisition of the written text and a multimicroprocessor system for real-time recognition of characters have been implemented. At present, the character recognition software is being transferred from the computer where it was developed to the multimicro structure [4].

Two different presentation methodologies are foreseen for the system, that is a paperless Braille display and synthetic speech.

In the future, the activity will be mainly devoted to the development of software for the interaction of the blind and for the control of complex formats in the input texts.

The same scanning and recognition system could also be used as an input peripheral in a computer-based paper Braille production system to be set up by the Regional Administration of Tuscany at the Florence Printing House for the Blind, with the technical support of the Special Project.

c) Paperless Braille systems

Paperless Braille has been considered, both for its use in the development of personal systems for the production of texts on magnetic supports and for the interaction of the blind with computers or with their environment (e.g. in schools).
A comparative test of commercially available systems has been performed at the "Davide Chiossone" Institute for the Blind in Genoa and a new equipment is under development by an Italian company (LACE Elettronica - Pisa), with the cooperation of the IROE (interaction and editing software) and the "Davide Chiossone" (specifications of functional requirements for the system). This is designed as a modular system which, with different options and peripherals, can be used in various contexts, both for personal and professional applications.

d) Graphics communication problems

An embossed paper plotter is under development at the IROE, for the production, with the aid of a computer, of embossed drawings to be used for testing different formats for the presentation of graphical information. It will be used to prepare drawings for applications in schools (in cooperation with a group of the Institute for the Blind in Milan) or as an output interaction and control means for a software studied to allow blind people to communicate graphical information to sighted people.

e) Low vision aids

A TV closed circuit system to be used as an aid for reading by low vision persons has been developed by an Italian company (LACE Elettronica), in cooperation with the group at the "Davide Chiossone". Two prototypes have been implemented, one of which was designed as a portable unit to be connected to a normal TV set, while the other was meant for a fixed installation. At present, their use is being evaluated at the "Davide Chiossone" and industrial production is being started.

f) Training for the use of the Optacon

This activity was essentially completed in the first Special Project, where a method for training children in the primary school to the use of Optacon was developed (Davide Chiossone).

g) Early education and rehabilitation: cognitive, linguistic, motor and emotional

The development and standardization of educational methodologies, rehabilitation models and testing procedures to be used in the period 0-5 years are considered in this research activity. Particular care is given to eliciting kynestetic and proprioceptive potentials (Davide Chiossone).

h) Mobility

Techniques for stimulating and eliciting kynestetic and proprioceptive potentials, to be matched to auditory ones, are under development and test (Davide Chiossone).

2) Main characteristics of the activity in the development of
   aids for the disabled

Some peculiar characteristics of the activity in the identification, design and production of technical aids for the blind
or low vision persons should be presented as an introduction to
the discussion.
The reintroduction of impaired people in a role which satis-
fies their needs of autonomy, from a practical as well as from
a psychological point of view, has different phases, such as:
a) quantification of the level of impairment and its medical
   causes;
b) functional rehabilitation and development of personal capabilities;
c) substitution or integration of the normal capabilities by
   means of aids;
d) reintroduction in society at a level which is matched to the
   capability level and the desires of the disabled.
Correspondingly, due to the fact that the very notion of
handicap as the difficulty to carry out an activity which is
considered normal in some contexts involves the interaction of
the disabled person with society [5], the problem of the development of aids has to take into account several factors, such as:
a) identification of the level of disability;
b) expectations of the impaired people;
c) acceptability of the possible technologies also from a psychological point of view;
d) an acceptable cost/performance ratio.
This means that, in the process of singling out the problems
and of identifying their possible solutions, it is necessary that
different disciplines cooperate in the task, and namely: medicine,
bioengineering, electronics, technology of materials, education,
psychology and so on. Moreover, it is also necessary to interact
with the final users of the aids and to accept their suggestions.
Another very important characteristic, which is useful to
point out in order to understand the difficulties of the research
and of the applications in this field is that, unfortunately, a
global aid is not available, at least for the completely blind,
and it is necessary to develop different aids for the different
tasks which have to be performed. Therefore, different aids have
to be thought up for the various applications and, in addition,
every aid should be matched to its different users.
This introduces difficulties in the choice of the appropriate

techonology and in the production, diffusion and maintenance of
technical aids, with a reduction in their availability and, unfortunately, an increase in their cost.

As a conclusion, in any research in this sector, once a problem has been pointed out in its general formulation, it is necessary to look for a technical solution which, at least, for aids
intended for personal use, complies with the following requirements [6]:
- technological and psychological practicability;
- flexibility of the approach and adaptability to the different
  users;
- portability;
- cost matched to the means of the users;
- availability in a short time and everywhere;
- serviceability, to avoid long delays in the repair procedures.
  Maintenance should be simple and reliability should be particularly looked after.
- ease of operation and care of ergonomic factors.

3) Microelectronics and aids for the disabled

The main impulse to the problem of the design and production
of aids for the blind and visually impaired comes, at present,
from the development of microelectronics, informatics and signal
processing techniques.

It is widely recognized that the present age in our society
is a transition from an economy based on manufacturing towards a
society based on creation, processing and distribution of information. If we consider, for instance, the labor force in USA today,
only 13% is engaged in manufacturing, while over 60% works one
way or another with information [7].

This fact has very important consequences in the field of
aids for visually impaired people from different points of view,
such as:
- the enormous impulse given to the microelectronics industry,
  with an obvious impact on the increase in complexity and the
  reduction of the electronic equipment costs;
- the great interest in all the technologies for the transduction
  of information to match its presentation format to the needs of
  different classes of potential users. This means that many technologies considered up to now only of scientific interest and
  used in practice only in the aids for disabled people, are now
  becoming interesting on a broader scale. A typical example is
  voice synthesis which is now being considered as a future general means for the interaction with computers. This technology,
  which is in perspective a low cost one being completely based
  on electronic components, will probably be available in the future with a large scale production.

These circumstances imply the possibility of an introduction of the visually impaired in the information world on an equality basis, if these efficient forms of information displays are really developed.

Obviously, in the "if" of the previous sentence lies also the main danger, which visually impaired people have to cope with. In fact, the information society could offer a unique possibility to reduce the gap between sighted and not sighted people, but it could also introduce a new form of segregation, if a suitable transduction is not provided.

The very important changes, which information and communication technologies are producing in society, require corresponding changes in the way of life of people in general, who have to switch from the use of tools to the use of information in computers through their peripherals. The possibility of reducing the gap between different classes of information users depends essentially on the generality and completeness of the approach to the study of methodologies for the transduction and presentation of information.

The specifications of the Japanese project towards the fifth generation computers, for example, seem focused in the right direction, considering the possibility of inputs in written form (character recognition) and voice (voice recognition), and of outputs in synthetic speech.

These developments, which have a very important impact on present changes in society at large, have fundamental consequences also for the development of the aids themselves.

To clarify this assertion let us briefly consider the general structure of a communication aid [8]. By definition, this is a system which transduces information to be transferred through a sensorial channel, which is still available. The general block diagram of such an equipment consists essentially of three blocks: an input for the information to be transduced (e.g. a stream of characters), the system used for this transduction, and an output for the presentation in a suitable format (e.g. synthetic speech). This is obviously the general block structure of a computer, where the CPU introduces the necessary intelligence to perform and/or to control transduction, and the matching to the different applications is obtained by using different input and output peripherals and a suitable software.

The main advantages which are reported in the literature for an information approach to the development of technical aids for the disabled are the following [9],[10]:
a) substitution of dedicated hardware, with a reduction in cost and an increase in reliability and flexibility;
b) use of complex information transduction means (e.g. voice for input and output), also taking advantage of the results in the development of techniques and hardware for signal processing;
c) inherent modularity of the implementation;

d) configurability of the systems to different situations with
   software modifications;
e) low cost of microprocessors;
f) high availability of commercial software;
g) transportability of the application software;
h) easy serviceability and availability of the systems.

As regards the disadvantages, the following ones are mainly
reported:

- low portability of microcomputer systems (but this situation is
  very rapidly varying, due to the introduction in the market of
  efficient portable systems);
- high power consumption (now reduced by using CMOS technologies);
- limited duration of standard models, due to technical obsoles-
  cence and/or to market reasons, and limits in present systems.

These observations are very interesting but they do not ex-
haust all the different aspects of the problem, by considering
only the substitution of the hardware in the aids.

The other aspect that must be considered very carefully is
the software to be run on the aids, whose cost and complexity, as
in all the applications of computers, could be in the future the
limiting factor of this approach. In fact, while it is easy to
write simple programs to implement some functions, which can be
used in the aids for visually impaired people, the development of
an integrated line of modular products with a reliable and easily
modifiable software is a problem of high complexity and cost.

Therefore, the standardization which is necessary to set up
a general structure for a communication aid, is essentially a
problem of choice of a software environment, which is general
enough to have a large hardware support and can guarantee an easy
transportability of the software and configurability of the system itself.

In summary, the following points have to be considered in the
development of integrated aids based on microprocessors:

- choice of a microprocessor chip, which has a good software support and a widely available operating system (e.g. 8080 and
  Z80 chips, with a CP/M operating system);
- choice of a standard, largely used hardware (bus and card format), where a very large number of interfaces is present, to
  obtain a good configurability of the system. The choice should
  preferably be made among products for the industrial market and
  not for the consumer market. Home and personal computers have,
  in general, a very low price in their base configuration, but
  they have also very severe limitations in the periphery expansion. Moreover, they normally present the very rapid obsoles-
  cence rythm of the consumer market, with a high risk of a dis-
  continued support of the products;
- choice of a high level programming language, which allows an
  easy transportability of the application software on different

134

types of hardware, and reduction to a minimum of the assembler
modules, which depend on the particular implementation of the
system;
- modular implementation of the software.
    However, microelectronics and informatics techniques will
certainly have a very important impact on the implementation of
aids for the disabled, according also to the following considerations for the implementation of technical aids.
    Three main approaches can be considered in this field [9]:
- implementation based on dedicated circuitry. In general, it
  is possible to have an optimized design but, due to the small
  market, the aids are expensive and of difficult serviceability;
- modification of standard equipment. This approach is generally
  more satisfactory, since it reduces the design costs and the
  implementation time. However, for the parts which are specifically designed, the same observations as in the previous case
  apply;
- use of standard equipment.
    The microprocessor approach to the development of aids can
allow an implementation obtained through the use of standard
equipment if, as it seems possible, most of the transduction techniques important in this field will become available in the future as general input-output means.

4) Use of new signal processing technologies

    Some care has also to be used, when the applications of new
signal processing technologies such as, for instance, speech synthesis, are considered. It is certainly true that speech synthesis
will be of fundamental importance in the aids for blind people,
and not only for them, for several reasons, such as the following:
- voice is a very natural way for information transfer, and also
  with very low quality synthesizers the learning time to obtain
  a good intelligibility is very short;
- voice is recognized to be a very efficient way to transfer information for general applications and very important research
  and development efforts are in process, with a foreseen increase
  in the efficiency of methods and a reduction in the cost of the
  related technologies (it is only necessary to look at the new
  products that almost every day are announced in the technical
  literature to be convinced of this);
- voice can be obtained with completely electronic means, without
  mechanical parts, which are often the limiting factor from the
  point of view of reliability and cost.
    However, it is not true that the existence and diffusion of
such techniques can automatically offer a solution to the problem
of the visually impaired. In fact, while most of the corresponding
commercial systems can be directly used in simple interactions as

the synthesis of alarms or of fixed sets of messages, when complex interactions, like the ones required for using computers or data banks, are necessary, specifically designed speech synthesis systems must be used, where an interaction is possible not only with the source of information but also with the synthesizer itself.

As an example of this assertion, let us consider a speech synthesis system to be used for the interaction of the blind with a computer. A list of desirable functions (which we reproduce from [7]) in this interaction system is presented hereunder. A talking terminal for the blind is considered useful, if this terminal:
- can instantly stop the voice on a word;
- minimizes hand movement when reviewing text;
- verbally announces error corrections;
- can adjust speech rate;
- provides sizeable review memory;
- verbalizes punctuation and special symbols;
- distinguishes between upper and lower case letters;
- identifies columns,
- can automatically spell unusual letter combinations;
- synchronizes print/voice;
- can expand letters to phonetic equivalent;
- can mark text for review;
- can skim read;
- can search memory;
- can say numbers as words;
- can supply personalized vocabulary;
- can redefine keyboard;
- can traverse tables;
- can pronounce unprintable computers characters;
- can suppress repetition characters;
- provides for an off-line preparation.

Moreover, all the above mentioned functions should be performed without any load on the host computer, which should be able to run its operating system and application software without any interference.

This means that the speech synthesizer to be used for the interaction cannot be one of the several cards, which can be inserted in standard microprocessors and, without important changes in the software, can be used only as output peripherals. There must be a microprocessor based equipment, whose software was studied for these applications.

This is the reason why we implemented the speech synthesis system as a microcomputer-based equipment. For simple interactions this system can be used as a peripheral of a computer with a suitable software driver. For general interactions, it can be connected, using two serial interfaces, between a computer and a

normal terminal, thus transforming it in a talking terminal for
the blind.

Finally, several new possibilities are in principle offered
by the integration of computers and telecommunication techniques,
which is generating networks for information transfer and new
services (e.g. teletex). Most of these networks connect data
banks, where the information is essentially presented in a coded
form. As a consequence most of the modern approaches to the production of printed material also start from the preparation of
texts in a coded form for the successive printing of them. For
example, modern newspapers are produced in this way, using remote
terminals. The availability of the coded form of texts could
solve the problem of the access of the blind to them, through
suitable output transduction means (Braille, synthetic speech),
if an easy interconnection with these networks is made available.

References

[1]   G. Castellini, P.L. Emiliani, P. Graziani, S. Rocchi, A.
        Tronconi, R. Vanni: "A Voice Synthesizer for Blind-Comput-
        er Interaction", Proc. IV F.A.S.E. Symp. on Acoustics and
        Speech, Venice, April 1981.
[2]   G.L. Francini, G.B. Debiasi, R.D. Spinabelli: "Study of a
        Minimal Speech-Reproducing Unit for the Italian Speech",
        JASA, 36, 6, 1968.
[3]   G.A. Mian, F. Morgantini, C. Offelli: "An Application of
        the Linear Prediction Technique to Efficient Coding of
        Speech Segments", 1976 IEEE Int. Conf. on Acoustic Speech
        and Signal Processing, Philadelphia.
[4]   A. Da Ronch, R. Spinabelli, C. Pagura: "An Optical Charac-
        ter Recognizer", 3rd Congr. on Medical Information, Europe,
        Toulouse, March 1981.
[5]   Office of Technology Assessment of the U.S. Congress (OTA),
        "Technology and Handicapped People", U.S. Congress,
        Washington, May 1982.
[6]   H.J. Blaszczyk: "Computing and the Handicapped: the Chal-
        lenge in Education", IEEE Computer, Jan. 1981, 15-17.
[7]   AA.VV.: "Voice Output for Computer Access by the Blind and
        Visually Impaired", Aids and Appliances Review, The Carrol
        Centre for the Blind, 8-10, Summer and Fall 1983, 1-59.
[8]   W. Myers, "Personal Computers Aid the Handicapped", IEEE
        Micro, Feb. 1982, 26-39.
[9]   G.C. Vanderheiden: "Practical Application of Microcomputers
        to Aid the Handicapped", IEEE Computer, Jan. 1981, 54-61.
[10]   G.C. Vanderheiden: "Computers Can Play a Dual Role for
        Disabled Individuals", Byte, Sept. 82, 136-162.

DESIGN AND EVALUATION OF AIDS FOR INTERACTION WITH A COMPUTER BASED
INFORMATION SERVICE

R.W. King
Department of Electronics and Information Engineering
University of Southampton, Highfield
Southampton SO9 5NH, United Kingdom

1. INTRODUCTION

Access to interactive computer systems is now a commonplace in
education, business and leisure. The growth of these
electronics-based information systems brings opportunities but
also threatens older, established practices. Disabled people,
in particular, may be disadvantaged by the rate at which
obselescence can now occur. In this paper, however, we discuss
some of the opportunities of information technology and
describe aspects of the design and evaluation of equipment to
give blind people direct access to interactive information
systems such as Videotex.

Our work has concentrated upon the design of non-visual
terminals based upon dynamic Braille and synthetic speech. We
have not studied the use of Optacon or any image enlargement
methods, although many of our findings would be relevant to the
use of either of these. We have chosen to use existing Braille
display and commercial speech synthesiser systems. The prime
focus of the work has been the provision of suitable hardware
and software to form interfaces between the Braille and speech
output devices and the information source. These interfaces
have to include features related to the content and nature of
the source information, as well as provide physical inter-
connections between the source and the 'display' devices.

Videotex is the type of information service considered in
detail. This allows users to access centrally-held data bases
via the telephone network. The information can be displayed on
a conventional TV receiver, and the user interacts with the
system by means of a simple dialogue using a 10 numeral,*,#
keypad. Since the introduction of British Telecom's Prestel
service in 1979, broadly similar services have developed based
upon compatible transmission and display standards [1]. Full
keyboards are now generally provided for user terminals to
enable message services and computer programme interchange to
be conducted, although the simple keypad described above
continues to provide the basic means of user interaction.

Dynamic Braille displays are, of course, well established for
professional computer interaction and for personal notes, etc.,
but they are expensive. Synthetic speech devices are now well
known and used in many products for blind and sighted people.
The object of this paper is to discuss how these two forms of
output can be incorporated in low cost non-visual Videotex terminals, and to discuss how their performance can be evaluated.

2. DESIGN CONSTRAINTS AND DESIGN STRATEGY

The output terminals and the Videotex source impose a number of constraints upon the design. These, taken together with the aim of low-cost solutions capable of operating in near real-time, lead to a three-stage design procedure which also has merits for the processes of evaluation. The constraints are presented first.

2.1 Output devices

Dynamic Braille and synthetic speech are essentially 'linear' output media. In the former, simple or contracted Braille data is presented under user control to the single row of cells, typically 20-48 in number, and the display is refreshed with new Braille when required.

The listener to synthetic speech has less control over the output. Speech is ephemeral: the listener has to adapt to the pace of the utterance and only by interrogative conversation can an utterance be 'replayed'. Natural though speech is for information gathering tasks, it tends to be used as an adjunct to visual material. We may anticipate that synthetic speech is not likely to be ideal for the output of information systems such as Videotex quite irrespective of the quality and intelligibility of the synthetic speech itself, although to an extent the shortcomings can be overcome by giving the user appropriate controls over the utterances. In order to achieve the capability of unlimited vocabulary output the synthesisers used here are formant-based vocal-tract models driven by phoneme codes.

Both displays require the source text to be translated into appropriate forms, and the translation processes into Braille and phonemes form part of the interface software.

2.2 Videotex

Our objective of low-cost implies minimal modification to existing Videotex terminals, thereby allowing our interface to be simply added-on. This turns out to be quite straightforward as it is possible to access directly the incoming data from within the receiver. We propose to use the normal Videotex terminal keypad (or full-keyboard where fitted) for page requests, and other normal Videotex system requests.

The display characters and the two-dimensional layout of the Videotex pages, on the other hand, present potential problems. The displayed characters are either alphanumeric (essentially ASCII) or graphical (3×2 matrix), and are used to form pages of 24 rows of 40 characters. A number of layout features have been identified [2] as having significance for the present application. These are continuous text, alphabetic graphics, pictorial graphics, multiple columns, tables, and indexes of list and sentence forms. Most pages possess two or more layout features.

An early decision was to discard graphical characters from further consideration, even where these characters are used to form words. The 'linearisation' of the remaining material takes into account the layout types in the manner described in section 4.

The final aspect of Videotex which demands attention is the 'interactive' or 'response' page type. These pages are provided for ordering and booking services and are no less valuable for blind than for sighted people. The sighted user is prompted to supply a suitable keypad response to specific questions indicated in turn by a flashing cursor. The non-visual terminals need to incorporate a facility to allow responses of this type.

2.3 Design Strategy

The interface design can be divided into three separate stages:-

reformatting : to convert the page layout into a suitable form for linear display.

translation : to convert the reformatted text into suitable Braille or phoneme codes.

output : to present the material to the user in dynamic Braille or synthetic speech and provide suitable user controls.

This division of the interface has two merits. Firstly, it is evident that the reformatting process required is the same for both forms of output. Secondly, it allows design and evaluation of the stages to be carried out independently, thereby allowing detailed knowledge of the system's shortcomings to be obtained, and giving greater insight into means of improvement.

The design and evaluation work has been conducted on a microcomputer development system, with the ultimate aim of incorporating the required hardware and software in suitable units together with the Braille display or synthetic speech devices.

3. EVALUATION CRITERIA

The evaluation of aids is always difficult. In the present instance we are exposing blind people to new display media and confronting them with a new type of information source. If the system works at all satisfactorily then a likely response is "when will it be available, and how much will it cost?" Long term market trials eventually, of course, yield the best answers, but in the meantime designers need to know whether the path being followed is sensible.

We have tackled this problem in a number of ways. Firstly, a blind user, an experienced programmer, gave periodic advice about a number of issues, particularly relating to the display controls. Secondly, as we shall explain in more detail later, we have evaluated the reformatting, translation and output

control stages independently, and outside the context of
Videotex interaction. Thse evaluations are partly objective,
and partly subjective. Finally, we have compared the performance of the non-visual Videotex terminals with that of
normal visual use of Videotex, with a particular view to
determining the 'efficiency' of our terminals.

4.   REFORMATTING AND ITS EVALUATION

The reformatting process is required to identify the page
layout features listed above and then present the textual
material to the translation stage in a suitable order.   The
identification task is a straightforward one in pattern
recognition which is aided by the use of colours in the normal
display. The colour background and character display codes are
processed in the reformatting stage to give a rough 'blocking'
of the layout components. The blocking is then tidied up by
infilling incomplete boundaries and removing small blocks.
Graphics blocks are removed at this stage. The second stage of
the process is to examine the character content of each block
in turn and classify it as continuous text, multiple column or
tabular.   This is done by scanning the rows and columns of
characters for spaces and numerals, a process which itself
permits   further blocking within, say, a multiple column
layout. Finally the blocks are assigned a type marker and order
marker.   The latter is based on a left-to-right, top-to-bottom
scan.

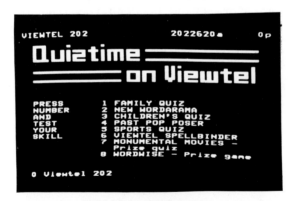

(a) Original page

(b) Reformatted page displayed on a VDU

Figure 1   An example of page reformatting

Figure 1(a) shows a typical page containing a title formed from graphics characters and a multiple column format. The automatically reformatted version in Figure 1(b) shows the removal of the title and the resolution of the two columns into a single line of text, and a list index. The *B*, *U*, *P* markers show where the formatter has inserted end of block, line and page markers.

In order to assess the effectiveness of the reformatting procedure a sample of 200 pages of British Telecom's Prestel service was processed. The resulting layouts were examined carefully, and the reformatting performance was categorised as:-
  perfect: correct reformatting and block/line marking
  imaged: page effectively unformatted-line markers only
  mixed :   some perfect, some imaged blocks
  disordered: incorrect reformatting, ambiguous result.

Table 1 shows the results for four types of page. The sample sizes reflect approximately the relative proportions of those types of page in the Prestel service.

Page Type	Index	Text	Tables	Multiple Column
Sample size	100	60	20	20
Perfect	80%	80%	100%	60%
Imaged	19%	10%	--	15%
Mixed	1%	10%	--	--
Disordered	--	--	--	25%

Table 1 Reformatter Evaluation

The reformatter thus works constructively on most pages - it may fail to do a perfect job for some but it is only the 25% of 10% of the pages where it introduces disorder. For these cases it is desirable to allow a blind user to have recourse to the unformatted source page. Tables are left unchanged from their original form, accounting for the 100% perfect performance.

5. TRANSLATION STAGES AND THEIR EVALUATION

5.1 Braille Translation

It was regarded as essential to provide a fast contracted Braille translator as well as one for simple Braille, in order to satisfy most users. The translation provided here is a compromise between accuracy, speed and memory requirement. All standard English contraction rules [3] are stored, together with a dictionary of the most common words in contracted form.

The algorithm attempts to minimise contracted word length, a process which can lead to 'illegal' contractions for long and relatively uncommon words. At the time of writing we have examined the translation/contraction accuracy for the 4000 most common words in English. 98% of these are contracted correctly while most of the remaining 2% are described by a Braille reader as incorrect but readable. In order to reduce the disturbance of miscontraction our display allows recourse to Grade I output at any time. The Braille readers who evaluated the system regarded this practice as acceptable, it being one which is possible only with a dynamic output. The translation algorithm (including the dictionary) occupies 8 kbytes of memory and operates faster than the output is transferred to the Braille display itself.

5.2 Translation to Phonemes

The synthetic speech conversion system contains a two stage translation process. The first stage is a text-to-IPA (International Phonetic Alphabet) translator while the second stage maps the IPA codes into the appropriate codes to drive the particular synthesiser device being used. The text-to-IPA rules are based on those of Elovitz [4] and are arranged in a data structure such that a character and its surrounding sub-strings may be matched rapidly to the appropriate IPA string, which is inserted into a buffer. When this buffer contains the phonemes for the required speech segment, such as a sentence or line of text, the phoneme codes are converted into the form for the synthesiser.

Synthesiser quality and intelligibility depends on the accuracy of the text-to-speech rules as well as the intrinsic nature of the synthesiser model. The translation is performed at a word level and consequently the output synthetic speech utterances contain no prosodic features of rhythm, pitch and stress that contribute to natural human speech.

A number of experiments with blind and sighted subjects has been conducted to gauge and compare the intelligibility of two synthesiser units. One result of these experiments which is of interest here is learning time. It took on average 40 minutes to improve the initial 50% word accuracy score to 95% for both blind and sighted groups of subjects.

The text-to-IPA rules have been developed to provide accurate phonemes for the 7500 most common English words. It must be reported however, that the translation of names, which tend to occur frequently in Videotex systems, is often rather poor. The text-to-speech rules occupy about 40 kbytes of memory and operate in less than one second for a 20 word speech segment.

6. OUTPUT STAGES AND OVERALL EVALUATION

6.1 Braille Display Length

Of considerable importance is the Braille display length, for the cost of such displays is largely dependent upon the number of cells in the row. We were fortunate to have a Clarke & Smith display strip of 48 cells made available for this work. In order to determine whether an optimum length could be found, experiments were conducted with 8 Braille readers, reading purely textual material in uncontracted Braille. Although the absolute speed ranged widely, corresponding to the individual's basic Braille reading speed, it was found that more than 3 words or about 20 cells does not significantly increase Braille reading speed. Figure 2 presents data from these experiments. The absolute reading speed attained by any individual is about half his normal Braille speed, a reduction which is due partly to having to activate the refresh and wait for the row to be set up with new Braille, and partly to using uncontracted Braille.

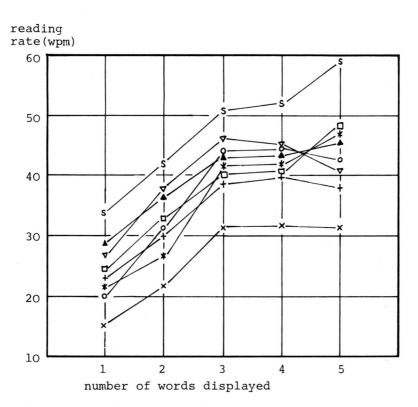

Figure 2   **Reading rate for 8 Braille readers against number of words displayed.**

6.2   Videotex Evaluation Experiments

Rather than use a set of pages selected from a 'live' Videotex service, most of the overall evaluation was performed on a graded set of pages created for the purpose and stored on a limited access basis on Prestel. The following tests explored

144

the use of the principal page types:
1. Use of a single index page
2. Use of two levels of index pages
3. Use of three levels of index pages
4. Reformatted multiple column page
5. Unformatted multiple column page
6. Timetable page
7. Interactive page
8. Free-run on Prestel.

Each test required the subject to determine a particular piece of information. For example, the timetable was used to find the departure time of a train required at a given destination before a specified time. The free-run on Prestel was used to determine a foreign currency exchange rate.

Four groups of subjects participated, designated as follows:-
SV: 4 sighted users of visual Videotex
SS: 9 sighted users of synthetic speech
BS: 8 blind users of synthetic speech
BB: 8 blind users of Braille

The subjects answered a short questionnaire on various aspects of the system.

6.3 Results

Two measures of performance are of interest. The first is accuracy, or success in finding the required information, the second is the time taken to complete each task.

(a) Accuracy
The four groups performed equally well, and perfectly, in tests 1,2,3,4,6, and 7. In test 5, using the unformatted page the groups scored as follows:-
SV: 90%; SS:50%; BS:50%; BB:30%
These results confirm the need for reformatting.

(b) Times taken on tasks 1-7
The times vary quite markedly between the groups, and between the tasks as shown in Figure 3. As anticipated, the synthetic speech terminal was the most time consuming to use. On average the time taken to access Videotex via Braille is 2 times that of visual access, while synthetic speech access is 4 times slower.

(c) The free-run experiment on Prestel.
This experiment revealed the complexity of the searching task on a Videotex system, and the difficulty of using a linear output media. Although the blind subjects were able to obtain the required information with similar time **ratios** as found in the previous tasks, **absolute** times of up to 35 minutes in the synthetic speech case may lead one to question the viability of such a system for routine, everyday use. The problem is that of memorising on-route indexing information. The use of keyword searching would be a major advantage but is not available on simple Videotex systems.

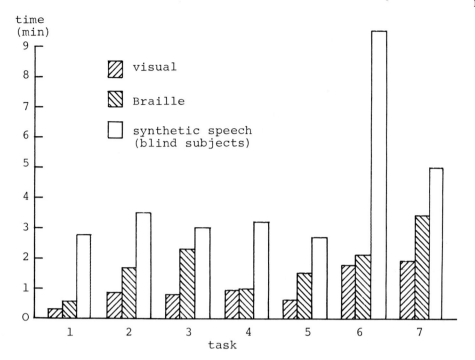

Figure 3. Average times for three groups of subjects to execute tasks 1-7.

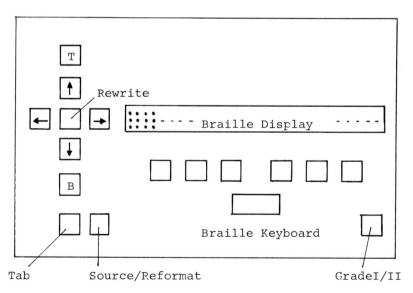

Figure 4. Proposed layout for Braille display controls. (Continuous use of the → key reads through the page)

6.4 Display Control

The Braille display controls must allow easy movement of the display window up and down, thereby effecting simple reading of tabular formats.   In addition, the tab marker allows rapid recall of a particular row, such as the table headings.   This has been effected by the inclusion of a standard 7-key Braille input keyboard.   Additional controls move the display window to left and right, rewrite the window and move the window to the page top and bottom. Grade I/II selection and reformat/source keys complete the controls. A proposed layout is shown in Fig. 4.

For the synthesiser it is necessary to provide controls to reduce the utterance down to phrase, word and spell levels from the root sentence or line modes.   This helps the user to overcome some of the limitations of the poor speech quality, and pace the speech output. Repeat, previous utterance, top and bottom of page controls are similar to those for the Braille display. The arrangement of these keys is less critical than that required for the Braille display. Further investigation is needed to determine the value of more sophisticated control to aid scanning of tables etc.

7.   CONCLUSIONS

This detailed study of non-visual output for Videotex has shown that both dynamic Braille and synthetic speech are technically viable and potentially useful for blind people. Careful consideration of the design stages and means of evaluation has led to what is believed to be designs which approach the optimum in terms of ease of use. The access times, compared with normal visual access are in some instances large, but not necessarily prohibitive, and the standard of presentation of the Videotex material after reformatting and translation is sufficient for Videotex material to be accessed accurately.

For both Braille and synthetic speech output imperfections in translation may be compensated by provision of suitable control functions, such as recourse to Grade I Braille and word spelling in the case of the synthesiser. Similarly an imperfect and practical reformatter is greatly aided by the facility to translate and present the source pages unformatted, but with graphics removed.

The synthetic speech output is less satisfactory, but for the large number of blind people who are unable to read Braille, synthetic speech is viable, and with improving quality will become more so. The potential of keyword searching, already a feature of many Videotex systems, is particularly advantageous for this form of non-visual output.

These displays can form the core of non-visual terminals for blind people. We then envisage means to interface, via suitable software, other types of source material for which different formatting, for example, would be provided.

8. ACKNOWLEDGEMENTS

The author wishes to acknowledge the work of N. Cope and Dr. O.R. Omotayo, as well as the financial support of the SERC, British Telecom and Clark and Smith Ltd and thank Mr. Brian Payne and all the blind and sighted subjects who participated in the experiments.

9. REFERENCES.

[1] Clarke, K.E., International Standards for Videotex Codes, Proc. I.E.E., Vol.126, No.12, (1979), pp1355-1361.

[2] Cope, N. and King, R.W., Conversion of Teletext and Viewdata into Braille, Proceedings of the Man-Machine Systems Conference, IEE Conf. Pub. No. 212, (1982), pp.196-200.

[3] Standard English Braille, Royal National Institute for the Blind, London (1971).

[4] Elovitz, H.S., et.al., Letter to Sound Rules for the Automatic Translation of English Text to Phonetics, IEEE Trans. ASSP, 24, 6, pp446-459.

DISCUSSION

Werner (to Doove)

I am referring to your last remarks on future development. You
indicate a development of a compact way of storing information
in audio or Braille format. Do you think of just storing spoken
books or do you also envision the possibility of storing texts
in inkprint to be converted when actually needed either to Braille
or spoken output? In the latter case may I also ask: are there
good quality output devices for the Dutch language? As compared to
English the output of German is comparatively easy but nevertheless
the output sounds rather monotonic with respect to the speech melody and furthermore the machines known to me so far have usually
some "foreign accent". How do you feel about this development and
what do you know about speech output in Dutch?

Doove

What I meant was storing spoken information (talking books) in a
digitalized way on a compact-disc. The output is not synthesized
speech but the natural human voice. Of course it is possible to
translate digitalized information to synthesized speech and in that
case it should be possible to store about 100 hours on one compact-
disc. I think that in the Netherlands some projects on synthetic
speech are on-going but the library for the blind has nothing to do
with it. As far as Braille-output is concerned, that's possible on
a compact-disc as well. In that case you need a paperless Braille
reading device.

Werner

This would be the next step. If you could do this, you could even
compactify things more or not?

Doove

I think that another problem is solved when the compact-disc is
used for Braille-storage and that's the problem of the voluminous
character of Braille on paper; I mentioned that in my speech. This
applies particularly to dictionaries and encyclopaedias. I think
that it is unfortunate just now that we cannot include people working in this field into those discussions. Another activity that's
coming up in August is the international Expert Meeting of the
IFLA Section of Libraries for the Blind, in Amsterdam. There I
will present a paper on the compact-disc as a possible carrier of
talking books. When the working group I told you about will be
established, then we can investigate the possibilities of this new
feature and that's what we are aiming at.

Tronconi (to Granstrom)

We know that some speech synthesizers are now available as indus-

trial products. Many of these devices as, for example, the Apple
speech card and the Commodore speech synthesizer, are very cheap.
I would like to know your opinion about the possible benefits
that the use of these devices can produce for blind people. In
particular, is it possible to work on the software to allow a
real interaction of the blind with computers using these devices?

Granstrom

There is a short answer to that and that is "no". But I could try
to explain why. These cheap devices are hard-wired, so that they
work on a fixed inventory of speech sounds. That means that it is
impossible to put any quality in them by software manipulation.
There is also the question if the speech quality is essential. In
some reports you see that the quality is not an issue at all. I
think that is wrong, in general. It is true that you can put up
with almost anything. If the blind are not able to read Braille,
something is much better than nothing, but if you use low quality
synthetic speech with lengthy material it might be very tiring.
The other thing is intelligibility. If it is low, it means that
you have to devote too much of your mental capacity actually de-
coding a message. Several studies indicate that there is quite a
difference between high and low quality speech.

Heyes

It is not really a question, but I think you might be quite amused
to hear of an application of synthetic speech to help blind people,
which is being tested in England at the moment, and that's the
talking "bus stop". The idea here is that the bus will pass over
a detector in the road, a hundred meters down from the bus stop,
and the bus stop will say "Ding-Dong - the number 6 is now approaching", and the visual handicapped person can then put his
hand out. In addition to that, the bus stop has a button which
when pressed the bus stop will announce the time of day, the
buses that use the stop, and the time of arrival of each. The
speech quality is extremely high but, of course, only a certain
number of messages are required, so it is not like your system
at all.

Granstrom

There are several applications of that kind using human speech,
coded, compressed, but still human speech.

Werner

I was just wondering, how can you modulate the intonation in your
system?

Granstrom

What we generally do is to try to derive where the stresses are

in the sentence and then use some general idea how sentence intonation is manifestly dependent on syntax and punctuation. It
is language dependent, and in the systems like this it will
also be rather stereotyped, because the machine doesn't understand what it is talking about. It will produce a neutral reading of the text, which might be good sometimes, or bad sometimes.

Emiliani (to Granstrom)

I would like some comments from you about the problem of the
quality of the speech. There was a first generation of synthesizers whose quality was very low, and in some cases also intelligibility was very low. Now we have a better quality, and in the
future we will have probably very good quality speech synthesizers, mainly if speech synthesis will be used for general applications, and therefore for a large market with very high invest-
ments in research and development. What I would like to know from
your experience is how you can measure quality in this kind of
applications. In general, quality is measured having listening
groups and asking people how they judge the voice in comparison
with the human voice. The quality is good if the voice is very
similar to the human voice, otherwise it's not good. One could
also consider another point of view: the voice is a code and,
even if we speak in one particular way, probably that's not the
only way you can organize a code for communication with voice.
Therefore, in some particular applications, you could also use
some different criteria for quality. You could try and develop,
let's say, some kind of artificial vocal code, which could be useful in some particular applications with a cheaper implementation.
Some tests were made in Italy for the Italian language and it was
found, for example, that a monotonous speech was more intelligible than a non-monotonous one with an artificial intonation.
Therefore, in some cases, for example in interactions which are
not very long, you could prefer a monotonous speech, rather than
a speech which is not monotonous, but which has a non-perfect
intonation.

Granstrom

You are touching on the problem of how much analysis do you have
in the system. If you have a very competent linguistic analysis
of the input texts, then you have a lot of information to carry
over the synthesis part of the system. But if you can't do the
analysis, if you are wrong in a lot of instances, then it might
produce misleading results, and in that case it might be better
to use a more neutral pronunciation. I think it's a short cut,
it's something you shouldn't aim at, because people usually communicate by speech and are so used to that code - it's a "de facto"
standard. I think it would be very hard to teach anyone a different auditory code that would be equally efficient. In the ex-

periments you were mentioning I guess that the implementation of
the intonation was actually very bad. We have made some experiments exactly in that area, trying to look at the intelligibility and naturalness with different approximations to the fundamental frequency, and it is very apparent that naturalness and
intelligibility go hand in hand. If you have a good intonation
contour, the intelligibility will be higher.

Emiliani

The working situation, for example, in the field of visually
impaired people is completely different from the situation in
which the tests are made. When you make a test of intelligibility, what you aim at is a general application. You say some
sentences and you want that most of these sentences are recognized, and at once. But, generally, when you are working in some
particular applications with disabled people, you can have a
training with that particular kind of voice. In some cases, you
find that the disabled, after training, are able to accept some
defects in the voice, because they get used to them. It's the
same situation when you have a friend who has a bad pronunciation, a defect of some kind. After some hours, you are able to
understand everything he is saying and you don't notice that he
has that defect. There is some kind of accomodation of people to
different codes. Therefore, this should lead, at least in particular situations, to a reduction in the equipment complexity.
Obviously, in ten years, for example, if we are able to have a
cheap and very high quality synthesizer, that would be the best
solution. But probably between the Votrax synthesizer and the
very high quality synthesizers, there could be some medium-qual-
ity ones which could be very useful in these applications.

Granstrom

Of course, I agree with your first point, that people have the
ability to adapt to different kinds of speech very rapidly.
I mean, often the situation is like ours, in this meeting. We
are trying to speak English and everyone is doing that in a different way. We have to adapt to the different versions of the
English spoken here, and that's not so hard. This is the only
possible way for us to communicate. But you couldn't draw the
conclusion that, since that's the case, all the English synthesizers could sound like anyone of us, trying to speak English.
I mean that we should aim at very high quality. I don't think
that the hardware is a problem any longer. That's my attitude.
It's better to try to aim, at the present time, at the best
available synthesizers. Because if you manage to get volume on
that kind of production, rather than something specialized for
the blind applications, then you get also the component price
down. You have the possibility to make the manufacturing effi-

cient, you can package things much more efficiently.

Emiliani

I was not saying that we have to be content with low quality.
I was only saying that there is a lot of debate about this problem at present, and some people say that speech synthesizers are
not high quality now and, therefore, they are not useful. I was
mantaining that probably even if they are not high quality, they
can be useful. If you can have better, and we hope to have better
synthesizers in the future, I think it will be better. But I
don't agree with people who say that synthesizers are not perfect, and therefore they are not useful.

Granstrom

I certainly agree with that. You shouldn't wait for the perfect
synthesizer. I think it's very essential that you get these things
out to the blind community for evaluation and for application.

Levett (to Granstrom)

I have a second order question in terms of radio and telephone
links reading out from a data base. Obviously, at the end of the
line, the selectability that you are building into your system is
different if you are reading out from available books in a library or if you are producing a newspaper. At the end of the line
how do you code the information for selectability? I mean, political versus sports, information or local versus national or international news, if you are dealing with that kind of information
systems?

Granstrom

It's a very important question, I think. The selection is a main
problem, how to structure the material so that you can get an
easy access to it. There is a possibility, if you have seen the
teledata system, for example. If you manage to automatically
structure the information in the framework of the teledata system, then you might have a partial solution to it. One problem
of accessing data bases for the blind persons is that data bases
are structured in different ways, and with each kind we get new
problems. So, one way might be actually to have interface programs between these data bases and the teledata network.

King

I shall be talking about some of these things in my paper tomorrow on videotex and conversion into Braille and speech. But the
essence of the answer to the question that you posed I think is
that the keyword searching is not essential for the use of synthetic speech as opposed to numerical indexes normally provided
in the systems.

Levett (to Granstrom)

My question is: how was the material on you small aids transcription indexed for the benefit of the blind using it?

Granstrom

In fact, this small aid is divided according to headlines and there are about a hundred of these headlines, that's the subdivision. If you want to know anything about used cars from 1970 to 1974, for example, that's one headline, say number 35. They are ordered sequentially. Then you know if you are at 31, you should move on. It's a very straightforward and simple indexing, in that case.

Tronconi (to Granstrom)

What is the price for the Italian text-to-speech version?

Granstrom

The price, I think, is around 2 thousand dollars for the stand alone system. There is no charge for individual languages, I think. It is equipped with the language that you need. What is interesting is that there is an ongoing development hardware-wise now. Infovox has an expansion card for the IBM-PC and compatible personal computers. There is also one version that has been built into other equipment such as the KURZWEIL reading machine.

Werner (to Soerensen)

I was wondering, perhaps you have some pictures of different fonts.

Soerensen

Yes, we have worked on recognition of isolated characters using several fonts.

Werner (to Da Ronch)

When you make this analysis for the alignment, do you proceed by going over the same page several times (with a multipass approach)? Can you store the full page for processing and then taking integrals of the blackening along the lines, until you find some blank columns?

Da Ronch

The first two steps of segmentations involve two different acquisitions. In the first step acquisition is made with a reduced resolving power, that is not with a pixel of 0.1 mm, but with pixels of 0.4 mm, four times greater. The sheet forms the basic memory store for the device every time it is necessary to scan it. In the second step, it is accessed by 2 cm high strips, and in each strip the line is looked for and the recognition is done.

Werner (to Da Ronch)

If you look at the topological structure of the letter set, how fine is your resolution? For instance, the letters D and O, and of course zero, have the same topological structure, but P and B should be already different. How fine is the resolution?

Da Ronch

The topological approach has a very high so-called rejection rate. The topological structure is present in the store, in the resident character, and then the unknown character may pass, or if it is not there, the image is rejected by topology. This rejection is rather high, over 10%, using the samples we have up to now.

Werner (to Da Ronch)

It could be used, possibly, just as a first diagnosis and then only in specific cases, depending on the topological structure, you would need just some key information to differentiate. So, for instance, I would think it is difficult to differentiate between D and O, because the difference consists just of a little corner.

Da Ronch

I believe that if no branch is in this D, the mistake is total.

Tronconi (to Bruel)

Do you think that it is possible to use speech synthesis as an output for your reading machine?

Bruel

In the first system the characters will not be read in order, because when the blind person is not able to understand the meaning of the sentence, he can go backwards. But for the second type of optical character reader, it is very interesting to consider the adding of a synthesized voice.

Question (to Bruel)

Can you say anything about the price?

Bruel

Delta will probably be manufactured at about 3 thousand dollars. I'm not able to give you a precise answer. It depends on the industrial partners.

Question (to Bruel)

Can you say anything about the reading speed with the Delta reader?

Bruel

The reading speed is only limited by the blind. The processor is very quick and is able to read at a speed of about 100 characters per second. For the first system, and not for the second. In the second, the speed is lower, because this speed is limited by the drawing table.

Werner (to Bruel)

I have possibly missed one point. How do you use the second system interactively?

Bruel

The idea is that it is very difficult to get a perfect system and, when the page has been read, the operator can control very quickly, on the screen, the whole page which has just been identified by the system, and he can correct the errors that have been made by the system.

Question (to Bruel)

How do you find the errors?

Bruel

The wrong characters appear in the video, they are brighter than the others.

Question (to Bruel)

How the machine itself detects the errors?

Bruel

When the machine is not able to recognize the character, it signals to the operator by flashing.

Soerensen (to Bruel)

When you have the classification results of the characters in a string of words, have you then tried to use contextual information in the error correction of the classified string?

Bruel

When the results are not very sure, the system prefers to flash the character, the wrong character.

Werner (to Bruel)

But I think you can trace the problem more generally. So far we have been concerned with the technical part of the talks we heard this morning. Now you can combine those devices with programming and a dictionary to see if the letters you have detected fit together in a plausible context.

Bruel

But it needs a very large software.

Werner

This is quite true. Its complexity is possibly comparable to that of the software we need for the translation phase, from inkprint to Braille.

Tobin

At the risk of appearing to be subversive of the whole aim of the conference workshop, or perhaps facetious at the very least, I would just point out that there already is an absolutely 100% optical character recognition device available. There is also, within the same device, an absolutely perfect, intelligible speech output component. These devices are in huge numbers (about 30 of them in this room at the moment), and in an age of growing unemployment, when large numbers of people in the de- veloped world are going to have a great deal of leisure, it might be an idea for engineers and psychologists to ask them- selves whether they are approaching the solution of the problem in an optimal way. The human being as a reader for blind people and others has a number of advantages: it is user friendly, you can alter the reading speed, you can do a lot of other things with it, and it may be that we ought to ask ourselves whether perhaps we are spending too much time, energy, and money on solving this problem in an engineering way. Some of us in this room have blind friends who are very skillful users of other human readers, and they can work for 5 or 6 hours with a relay of these readers coming in. All right! Too subversive, too fa- cetious, but just to remind ourselves that there are other ways of solving the problem.

Da Ronch

I know that one consequence of a visual handicap, as some blind men say, is the dependence on the instructors or other persons. This justifies the effort of making a machine which is far less perfect than a human being. This is done to assure a certain freedom for the blind in their access to written texts, that is to make them able to take the text themselves, to read the text themselves, to choose the text themselves, without excluding any other type of interaction with other people, who may see and read very well.

Spinabelli

May I also point out that a human being would be more costly than an automatic character recognizer? On the long run, I mean.

Levett

There are very good points on both sides of this particular
question. I think that one of the problems that we have to anticipate involves the organization of health care facilities in
general and for rehabilitation in particular. It's one of the
obvious aspects that comes from the use of technology. The hospital, in these past 20 years, has changed character, so that
today 30% of its functions deal with information and technology
and probably will go up to 50%. I think that with this in mind
we are faced with the correct kind of mix between the man/ma-
chine interface, and this is a very difficult problem. Obviously, we would like reading to others, whether it is to young
children or to blind friends. This is great, it is entirely within the human frame. There is of course the other side of the
coin as it has been pointed out, the question of dependence.
Sometimes the machine, hopefully in a human environment, is essential. In health care delivery, the question of whether the individual or patient is likely to tell a particular problem to a
human being (doctor), who has not been essentially trained in
dealing with any other problem than medical, is an important issue. It may be more appropriate and it has been demonstrated
that certainly some patients would tell the machine certain problems that they will not divulge to the doctor. This probably reflects the training in the medical profession as much as anything else as well as human behaviour. But obviously we have to
go to some kind of optimal system, the kind of mix necessary between technology and the human being and the man/machine interface. It's not an easy question or consideration, but one we are
faced with more and more.

Graziani

My opinion as a researcher and a user is that autonomy is a very
important point. To be handicapped means to depend on other persons. If one technological aid makes me able to perform some
tasks in an autonomous manner, then I'm not handicapped any longer.

Emiliani

I would like to make another comment. The question was why must
we invest a lot of efforts and also of money in developing character recognition and speech synthesis technology for use in this
field? But I think the situation now is not this one, that is
character recognition techniques and speech synthesis techniques,
and voice recognition techniques are being developed for other
applications and a very large market is foreseen for these systems. So, the problem now is not whether we have to invest money
and efforts in developing these techniques. In the next future,
they will be available for a very large market, and the problem

is how to use them in the field of impaired people, how to construct an efficient man/machine interface, and how these techniques can be integrated in the general problem of the rehabilitation of impaired people. I think that this point is very important because till some years ago the people involved in rehabilitation had to develop these techniques, and now these techniques are almost on the market.

Thomsen

A lot of electronic equipment is available to me as a sighted person, and I can use it or I can just leave it. It's commercially available to me, and it's up to me if I want it or not, or if I can afford it. I think that our age is going to create the same situation for the blind and visually impaired as well. I have three comments to make on the future developments of reading machines. I think that in your laboratories you should carefully consider three things. The first is that so far those machines we have seen on the market have been far too expensive. The second is the size. These machines are more or less stationary machines, office equipment, so that the blind user has to take the material to the machine in order to get it read. There should be a more portable machine, so that you can take the material and the machine with you to the library or whatever it is. The third thing is that the machines we have seen so far on the market are far too complicate to handle. They require more or less that you are a B.A. in mechanical engineering or a computer programmer, or a computer scientist to handle them. I think that for the KURZWEIL machines, it is necessary to know how to operate the keyboard, and this is not a reading aid for the ordinary blind user. So I think this point should be scrutinized carefully even when you develop your machines in your laboratory.

Silver

I like to agree absolutely with Dr. Thomsen, and also to some extent with my colleague, Dr. Tobin. I didn't see why we have to consider the use of people and the use of machines as alternatives. Surely, they are complementary. I have asked thousands of people who are registrable as blind, what it is they want to be able to do, and it is very rare to have two people who say exactly the same thing. I agree that what blind people need is independence, to be independent and autonomous, and this we must preserve because one of the main problems with using a reader is that you can't turn him off! But one of the main advantages of the reader is that it perhaps provides an old person with company and human contact. I don't see that because we are developing machines, that necessarily excludes us from amusing people, and also because we have people available that doesn't mean that there aren't people who would, like me, wish to wake up at 2 o' clock in the morning to finish a novel, and may not have a reader handy. Surely, we can use all of these things when it's appropriate.

Tobin

It really wasn't my intention to be subversive. I really wanted to do what, I'm sure, all of us have been doing privately, namely to remind ourselves that there is a variety of ways of solving problems and that it is easy for those of us who earn our living by working for the handicapped, sometimes to think that the way to do it is to provide them with autonomy by devices. We've got to have the right mix, haven't we? To take up Janet's point, we want to have access to the machine for a variety of purposes and at different times of the day. But I would want to mention the case of a professional blind man, and I'm thinking of one in particular who is a senior administrative officer. His way of tackling his reading problems, and he has a great deal of reading to do, is to get his secretary to look through the 50 letters that have come in that morning, and in half a minute - because that is what it will take - to say: "Ah, here, it is an important one, it is from so and so. I think we ought to deal with that first". In other words, the human reader can act, if you like, as a screening device before perhaps the blind reader puts the material through machine-readable form. I want to ask those of you who are engineers to bear in mind what is the rôle of the human reader in the whole system. I think there is really a danger that we will say that autonomy can only be provided by having devices. Yes, we can work on this, but I suggest that we are going to make people autonomous by getting the right mix. May I just conclude by saying I'm frightened of the kind of situation that I envisage occurring if we put everything onto machine systems. I know a blind boy of 16 who is at a school for the blind, and he spends his week-ends at home, and the whole of the week-end, from Friday evening to Sunday evening, is spent by him listening to his tape-recorder, doing things that involve him in a relationship with devices. When he is at school, he is forced to interact with other human beings. He spends the week-ends at home interacting only with machines. I don't think that this is good for his development. I think that he ought to be spending more of his time interacting with other people. None of us is autonomous, none of us, in any way! We have to encourage him to interact with other people. I think that the point is that we should regard dependence upon other people not as a limitation upon us. We are a gregarious species, by nature, after all, and I think we want to get the correct balance, and I would ask the engineers to keep this point in mind, and sometimes before they try to solve a problem, ask if there is already a mix available now that would allow the essential human contact to be maintained, and particularly when we come to children. I'm afraid some of our inventiveness would allow blind or deaf or physically handicapped children to do all their learning by machines. Socrates taught the slave boy Pythagoras' theorem by standing in front of him and drawing the signs with his ruler, and asking the boy "What now?" and the boy learnt because of that interaction between himself and the skilled teacher. I think he learnt more than Pythagoras' theorem when he was doing this. I think he learnt something about the interrelationships between people and how at one time you can be a learner and depending upon other people and, at the same time, you can then become a teacher and have others depend upon you. Because, after all, as researchers and educators and lecturers, we are dependent upon the people we are speaking to, just as they are dependent upon us.

Werner

Of course, I agree with you up to one point. If you are going to do fundamental research or development, usually you will not account in advance of what quality is absolutely necessary. Sometimes you have some objective that you cannot meet completely, but you try to meet it as good as possible. On the other hand, as I know from my own work in research, you go further than is actually needed for the special purpose. I think that in this kind of work we have not yet reached the stage where we can really judge what is absolutely necessary and how to achieve it most cheaply. In many cases we are curious how much we can achieve, regardless of the costs. Only in the second stage you try to make it economical. Some systems which are produced have not yet reached this stage. Economy will be reached on a production in a series of tens or hundreds. So, I mean, we should try to be honest in doing this kind of development, to provide some satisfaction to the researchers. I think we all know the satisfaction of having some result which you didn't believe was feasible. We shouldn't cut off this part of motivation.

Silver (to King)

I was interested in whether you considered the possibilities when you got the linearization stage, of putting your material into a VDU as large print. I've got the impression, and please correct me if I'm wrong, that your visual displays were the normal visual displays, they weren't in any way modified. It seems to me that if you've got the thing already stored in a linear form, you have a fantastic opportunity to reach a much larger group of the visually disabled, by giving a large print display. Have you considered this?

King

Yes, on an undergraduate project, I tried to do this particular

thing with the BBC micro, one of the cheapest available. Like
many undergraduate projects, it didn't come to the stage where
it could be demonstrated. But I'm glad of your encouraging
words.

Granstrom (to King)

I would like to have more details about these experiments, because we have carried out a similar kind of experiments. I think
there is a general observation that speech communication with
machines in the information retrieval tasks is very efficient.
The other thing is that I wonder if your linearization method is
actually necessary. I mean, the videotex medium is made to display information on a certain area, and the spatial information
could be used, if you supply more control for the reader. It
might be advantageous actually to keep the formatting of the page.
The comparatively low results that you get for speech synthesis,
I'm inclined to interpret that as an evaluation of the low quality speech. It is also likely that you haven't given the subjects
enough control over the reading of the page. In our experiments
it was extremely important to give the reader a lot of controls
to be able to move around on the page, find out the structure
of the page and pick up the important information.

King

I would agree that's the area which perhaps needs most attention.
On the linearization process, I think it is valuable because,
for example, when you take a multiple column page, you can image a joy-stick control to move up and down and around. I think
that the time taken would possibly be greater than that taken
for linearization, which in most cases makes a very good attempt
at producing sensible format for speech. I think pre-processing
is very valuable, although it is perhaps less so in the dynamic
Braille case, where suitably used controls can allow to go up
and down and across. I think it is essential for the synthetic
speech.

Granstrom

We think there is inherent worth in keeping the formatting that's
on the page. As a user of the system you will come back to pages,
and perhaps if you are frequent users, then you will learn the
layout of the page. There is also another question. How much
training did these people have in actually using the system, because I think they might show a heavy training effect for the different media, since speech is quite different from the page displayed. Braille is more close to it, speech synthesis might be
more sensitive to training, in this case.

King

I think there is more work needed on this. Our subjects were

162

"naive". They had practice of using synthetic speech for an
hour or so and a brief introduction to the keypad controls. But
essentially they were naive users, as videotex is supposed to
be a system which can be used naively, without intimate knowledge. In time, training of course helps. I'm sure that the excessive time taken by the synthetic speech listeners can be
shortened, I've no doubt about that. I think we would expect
about a factor of 2.

Tobin

I'd like to make a point and then I'd like to pose a question to
Dr. King and Dr. Emiliani. Of course, speech registration and
processing occurs over time. It has temporal aspects to it, whereas visual information has spatial aspects. Any information that
has a temporal aspect to it, is going to invoke cognitive factors such as short-term memory, whereas this is probably not such
an important factor with visually presented information which has
a spatial aspect. It seems to me, therefore, that any speech presented information is going to require the application of a short-
term memory capacity in the learner, and this may be accounted
against it when you are doing a comparison. Because, unless they
can keep re-hearing it, perhaps having information exceeding
their short-term memory capacity, a single presentation will present problems. Whereas if presented visually, the spatial aspect,
I would think, uses less short-term memory capacity and that may
account for the difference in visual and Braille reading, on the
one hand, and the understanding of speech on the other. You can
overcome it, of course, by re-presenting the material. But that,
of course, means that you are going to require time again. I'm
a great believer, in fact, in presenting information in as many
different forms as possible, to build some redundancy into the
system. But the question I'd like to pose to Dr. Emiliani and
Dr. King is: at what point do they think that the evaluation of
the systems should be handed over to people other than the in-
ventors? Dr. Emiliani made considerable reference to evaluation
and Dr. King also. With the device, you get a group of people who
are very committed to the success of the system. They become very
knowledgeable about the system and they are highly motivated to
make the system work. Now, in the long run, of course, the designer must hand over part of the evaluation procedure to somebody
who hasn't got an emotional commitment to the device. It is very
easy, I think, to raise the expectations of users by reporting
only one evaluation of it. I think one cannot ignore the fact
that you get a little group of blind people, the ones who are
first introduced to your device; they want it to work, they are
grateful for it. But, in the long run, when I want to confirm the
evaluation as a developmental evaluation. This problem has to be
addressed by the designers. Where do we build this in? Has it got

to be at the end of the line or there is any possibility of
building it into the system earlier?

Emiliani

I think that the evaluation should be made by completely different persons from the ones who have built the system. In fact,
in the special project we are trying to organize the evaluation
in normal working places, without our control. I must say that
I think the evaluation must be made by other persons, but it
must be done reasonably. It is not possible to give a synthesizer or another aid to a blind person and say: "Well, tell me
what you think about this". You must organize a training and set
up some methodology for the use and the evaluation of aids.
Then, at the end of this process, obviously, the evaluation must
be done by people other than the ones who have built the system
and are emotionally involved in the system itself.

King

I agree with that completely. One problem is that one needs the
money and a friendly manufacturer to provide for a trial involving enough independent disabled users. With only one or two
prototype models you can't go very far. But I agree with Dr.
Emiliani's remarks in general. Manufacturing seems to be a major
problem in this area.

Soede

I think we should be a little bit more specific on evaluation.
You can distinguish, probably, three levels of evaluation. First
of all, the technical evaluation. The engineers are making a
product and they have to evaluate if the product is technically
functioning as it was earlier specified. Second, the functional
evaluation: the product you have made, is it really working
according to the functional specifications, as they were when you
started the project; the testing is still in a laboratory environment with potential users and/or other people. Finally, the
field evaluation: this should be strictly performed by people
other than those involved in the design task. But the first stages
can probably be intermixed. Your lecture was a good example, I
think, of those first two levels of evaluation, done in order to
get a good product. Much of this evaluation, you can consider as
sorting out things for having more detailed specifications. You
can say it's evaluation, and at the same time it's also research
to be done to have a good product.

Levett

I'm thinking of relating biomedical engineering and the general
assessment which was given by Dr. Emiliani, to the problems that
occur, for example, in hospitals, where you have maintenance

teams being responsible for safety. Conflicts of interest and
bias are built into the system. Therefore, we have to develop
evaluation protocols, clinical trials, etc., to try to minimize
as far as possible the kind of bias or conflicts of interest
that can occur. I think the short discussion on the neurophysiological aspect of spatial/temporal processing is a rather
intriguing one, but I may add also the psychological concept of
divided attention, and whether we are dealing with the divided
attention problem or whether we are dealing with a neurophysiological problem of errors. Do we know enough about errors in
visual fixation mechanisms? I think that there are a number of
rather interesting problems of a basic neurophysiological nature
that have to be looked into.

Bruun

My point is that something could be done from the system side,
so that it can be adapted and be as simple as possible, to be
also used for synthetic speech.

King

Well, of course, one of the advantages of the synthetic speech
is that it does have a large potential market. However, I'm
doubtful whether information systems such as videotex can be made
sufficiently efficient in synthetic speech output for general
use, although of course a simplified data base such as one might
have in telephone answering systems, could be efficiently implemented in synthetic speech. Well, I think we can build on the
advantage for the potentially large market for synthetic speech,
but I think we need to take into account the particular problems
of visual disability in this case.

Bruun

In Denmark we have systems called telebanks, I don't know if
they are used in your country too, but we can dial on the digital telephone and the bank answers the question, and you find
how much you have to pay for taxes and so on. Do you have the
same in your countries? I mean, such systems could be improved
very much.

King

But they are quite restricted, I think, in terms of vocabulary
and then you can use a better quality of reproduced recorded
speech, and I think the level of complexity of the interaction
is quite low. It isn't as deep as going through a very large
data base such as videotex or perhaps using synthetic speech for
computer programming.

Werner

May be I could ask one simple question in this context. I don't

quite see the point why we really have to use videotex to transfer data such as they are digitized in some forms or characters
to blind people and then retranslate it. Don't we do things
twice? Originally videotex has to be organized, I guess, from
some material which was stored or produced in the usual way
that we could also use as input for books, for data, for printing, and so forth. I'm not familiar with videotex really. But
wouldn't it be possible to transmit the information in its input form, but not necessarily formatted? It's more compact, and
it could be easily handled directly.

King

That's correct, but someone has already paid for that process,
and this is available simply by pressing one button on your
videotex receiver, to receive this information already coded up
in that form. The other point, I think, is that videotex has been
considered something which can change very rapidly, like a daily
newspaper. So the information is only there on a very temporary
basis. If a very large proportion of users of this effectively
have paid for it all and we can provide a reasonable interface,
then we are in fact saving a lot of money, using very standard
transmission protocols which the telephone affords, these devices
afford. The other point, that perhaps I could add, is that the
standard protocols are now being used for transmission of a very
wide range of services, including computer programs, and many
domestic computers such as the BBC micro, the Acorn micro, and
so on, can be plugged directly into this transmission protocol.

Werner

I don't know the way videotex is produced, information or as a
"picture", i.e. formatted, etc.

King

Just information. Twelve hundred bits per second. The point is we
do not need the picture. But it is cheap. It's mass produced.

Spinabelli (to King)

I'm referring to your diagram in which it is shown that synthetic
voice listening can be four times as long as Braille output.
Did you make your experience with only one kind of voice?

King

With two synthesizers: Votrax and Microspeech.

Session 3: LOW-VISION (Clinical, Social, Psychological
 ───────── ───────── and Technological Aspects)

Chairman: D.H.A. Aberson

Organization of the Distribution of Low-Vision Aids
M. Warburg

Reading by the Elderly (Reading by Subjects with
Normal and Low Vision)
D.H.A. Aberson

Assessment of the Needs of Low-Vision Patients
J.H. Silver

Low Vision Aids and Some Perceptual Aspects of Reading
by the Partially Sighted
M.J. Tobin

Visual Impairment in Greece: Health Service Organization
J. Levett, J. Yfantopoulos, J. Tsamparlakis

Necessity of an Interface Between Research Output
and Social Needs
M.I. Campo, A. Testa

Discussion

ORGANIZATION OF THE DISTRIBUTION OF LOW-VISION AIDS

M. Warburg
The Copenhagen Eye Clinic for the Mentally Retarded
Gentofte Hospital
Denmark

Low-vision aids enlarge the retinal image either by
enlarging the object or by optical systems, telescopes
or lenses. While the majority of visually impaired people
prefer simple plus lenses, some will benefit from the
more complicated systems which are commercially available.
The problem is, that the dispensing of the aids has a
loose structure so that the technical development is
much in advance of the distribution to the consumers. A
number of strategies for dispensing visual aids are implemented concomitantly:

1. Selling over the counter in drug stores and other
   unprofessional shops.
2. Dispensing by trained optometrists or opticians.
3. Prescription by an ophthalmologist, dispensing by an
   optometrist/optician.
4. Prescription and dispensing in low-vision departments
   of major hospitals.
5. Community low-vision clinics.
6. Low-vision clinics run by organizations for the visually
   impaired.

Research and development

It is characteristic of the distribution of low-vision aids
that a close co-operation between research and development
(R&D) and dispensing is only rarely present. This is
interesting when compared to the fruitful interaction between

dispensing and R&D concerning hearing aids, and the explanation is probably that ophthalmology has been hesitant
to acknowledge the treatment of visually impaired people
as a subspeciality.

Demands

There is an increasing demand for low-vision aids in the
Western world because more people grow old and because
mainstreaming (integration) of visually impaired students
in local schools depends upon a wide range of technical
devices enabling the student to follow the curriculum of
the sighted, preferabling by using the same texts and other
educational materials. Organizations for the disabled demand
equal rights and claim that technical solutions to compensate
the impairments should be available whenever possible and
necessary. The organization of the distribution of aids to
visually impaired people requires an analysis of the requirements of the different groups of consumers.

Consumers

There are three main groups of people with low vision, viz.
1. The elderly
2. Educable children, adolescents and adults (employed or
   unemployed)
3. Multihandicapped children and adults

The elderly

About 46 per cent of all severely visually impaired people
reported (legally blind) are over 65 years of age (Goldstein
1973), but underreporting is a problem. Thus patients in

geriatric wards or residents in homes for senior citizens
do not have regular visual assessment.

The main causes of visual impairment in the elderly are
cataract, glaucoma and macular degenerations, and treatment
is available for a number of these conditions. Acquisition
of low-vision aids without an ophthalmological examination
is therefore unwise.

In most cases visual impairment occurs after the patients
have ceased gainful employment, and neither professional
rehabilitation   nor Braille reading skills are required.
The elderly usually demand low-vision aids that are technically easy to handle, they need simple motility aids and spoken
texts. Rehabilitation of activities of daily living (ADL)
will give them more years in their own home.

Senior citizens often have little information about visual
aids, and if they have, they find it difficult to travel to
special clinics where the aids are professionally prescribed
and dispensed. Their endurance is low, and dispensers with
little experience often feel disillusioned by the short
span of time in which the aids are used, because they are
unaware of the importance of being able to simply sort
reading materials (bills, letters, official papers) into
those that need immediate answers and those which can wait
for a relative to turn up and read.

The structure of the distribution of visual aids to the
elderly must therefore meet the following requirements:

1. The availability of the aids must be well advertised.

2. Minimum travelling to the location is essential.

3. Staff should comprise an ophthalmologist, an optometrist

and a social worker. Mobility training should be avaiable.

4. Close co-operation with an eye department to ensure the
   prompt treatment of observed disorders.

These requirements are easily met with if the low-vision
personel are members of the staff of a stationary eye
department. Minimum travelling could then be accomplished
by extensive use of taxi cabs or by housing the low-vision
personel in a specially designed bus (Henkind and Suarez 1974,
Brinck et al 1981). This bus could arrange regular visits to
geriatric wards, homes for senior citizens and other community
facilities for the elderly.

Educable children, adolescents and adults

Among all legally blind, 10 per cent are congenitally impaired,
while about 45 per cent of all blind or severely visually
impaired are 20 to 65 years of age (Goldstein 1973). In this
group of people the causes of the visual handicap are diverse,
many conditions can improve through surgical or medical treatment, some patients have associated disorders that need attend-
ence and about one half of the causes of visual impairment
in childhood and youth are hereditary. It is therefore common
for a school and a rehabilitation center for visually impaired
people to have their own eye clinic where the ophthalmologist,
the optometrist and the engineer have a close co-operation.
Students in the schools and rehabilitation centers demand
sophisticated aids, and teachers and technicians are trained
to teach how to use them. Rehabilitation officers can adapt
working places to suit a disabled person and many such centers
have close co-operation with R&D personel.

Children who are mainstreamed or integrated in normal schools
have less easy access to low-vision aids. In some countries
they are invited to yearly visits at the Blind School, in
others they are seen by local optometrists or ophthalmologists
who have little experience with the great number of disorders
giving rise to severe visual impairment. If mainstreaming
results in local rehabilitation new developments will reach
the consumers late.

People who become disabled after finishing their education and
vocational training need medical, technical and social advice,
and this is often unco-ordinated. While the elderly had
difficulties in travelling to the low-vision clinics, this
is not so for the young and mature disabled people, their
problem is that there are too few of these facilities and this
gives rise to an impressive waiting list.

The structure of the distribution of visual aids to young
educated in local schools and to mature people who loose
vision after some years of gainful employment must therefore
meet the following requirements:

1. Units well-spread over the country

2. A full assortment of visual aids

3. Staff comprising ophthalmologists, optometrists, engineers,
   social workers, teachers, and mobility instructors

4. Close co-operation with an ophthalmological and genetic
   department.

A low-vision department associated with a major hospital will
meet these requirements.

Multiply handicapped children and adults

Visual impairment among multi-handicapped persons is grossly

under-reported. Thus a screening for legal blindness among
mentally retarded children in Denmark (Warburg et al 1979)
disclosed that a third of the severely visually impaired
children had not been notified. The total number of legally
blind retarded children equalled the number of blind children
without intellectual problems, and the prevalence of severe
visual impairment was 200 times the prevalence in the
general child population. Ongoing investigations also indicate
that there are deaf-and-blind children among the mentally
retarded who have not been ascertained. In deaf-schools about
lo per cent of the pupils have moderate visual problems.
Even a mildly reduced acuity makes it very difficult to
lip-read, and progressive visual impairment unrecognized
in a child with hearing loss compromises vocational training.

About 10 per cent of visually impaired children have mild
to moderate hearing loss, the prevalence among adults is not
known. A hearing loss of 30 dB makes it quite difficult for
a visually impaired person to follow conversation.
The causes of visual impairment among retarded children
are many, and often represent rare syndromes, new syndromes
are continuously being described. Many of the causes are
hereditary and their identification gives an opportunity
for genetic counselling of the families. Cataract occurs in
many syndromes and can be operated, anomalies of refraction
are much more common among mentally retarded individuals than
in the general population (Woodruff et al 1980) and result
in unnecessary visual impairment unless glasses are prescribed
and used.

Among children with combined hearing and visual impairment

those who contracted rubella in foetal life are still the
commonest but unfortunately immunization is becoming
introduced in most countries. A substantial number of the
rest of these children have retinal degenerations which are
progressive, and the rest have rare syndromes.

Visual impairment among children with motor handicaps are
mainly due to optic atrophy, and many of these children have
also speech disorders. They communicate by Bliss, sign language
or learn to type, but in all cases visual impairment must be
identified to ensure that the children are not wrongly taken
to be mentally retarded.

Children with mental retardation, hearing loss or motor impairments are often educated in special classes even though these
may be located in ordinary schools. It is characteristic that
the staff has little knowledge about low-vision aids and even
spectacles and hearing aids may be difficult to introduce.
Since the demands of these children must be voiced be their
parent and teachers information has a high priority.

Most deaf-blind people have some residual vision and hearing,
many learn to use magnifying devices and some read Braille.
Children with motor impairment find magnifying aids difficult
to use because they are unable to keep the object in focus,
they benefit from spoken texts. Children with an intellectual
development below 2/3 of their chronological age will rarely
learn to use magnification, they have to go closer to the
objects, and this gives them serious draw-backs when they grow
old and presbyopic.   Spoken texts can be used by some, but

most of them use their tape-recorders for music.

Activities of daily life is difficult for a person with a
motor impairment if vision is also defective. This is
noted at the table, when dressing, at school and when
the patients propel their wheel-chairs under adverse
conditions such as in dim light, in unknown localities
or among obstacles. Technical aids would be of great
importance to solve this problem.

There are very few low-vision teams specialized in caring
for multihandicapped patients, the travelling distance to
such centers is long, and the multihandicapped persons are
difficult to assess when they are tired from travelling,
more-over these are patients who must be accompanied so
that expenditures become high. The structure of the distribution of visual aids to multihandicapped persons must therefore
 meet the following requirements:

1. Identification of visually impaired multihandicapped
   individuals
2. Information of parents and staff
3. Prescription of simple aids
4. Staff comprising ophthalmologist, teacher, mobility
   instructor, social worker and optometrist
5. Minimum travelling to the location
6. Close co-operation with an ophthalmological, genetic and
   audiological department in a major hospital.

The needs can be met by a low-vision staff with both stationary
and mobile facilities whose personel are staff-members of a
stationary eye department.

Discussion

Research and development of visual aids have been successful,
but there are a number of reasons why the visually impaired
people have restricted access to them, namely the lack of an
ophthalmological speciality in low-vision, the increase in
the number of elderly people, mainstreaming of visually
impaired children so that the schools for the blind are no
longer pivotal in looking after the needs of the legally
blind, the emancipation of the disabled resulting in their
voicing of their needs and lack of assessment of visually
impaired people with multiple handicaps.

Delivery of visual aids over the counter may result in
delayed treatment and is therefore unwise both from individual
and socio-economic aspects. The large number of individually
rare disorders and the wide range of visual aids require
that the low-vision unit has a reasonable number of patients
so that experience can be gained.

Delivery of low-vision aids and other services to visually
impaired people depend upon multidisciplinary teams wherein
the ophthalmologist, the optometrist, the teacher and the
social worker are equally important. The service of an
engineer and a technical work-shop must be available. Cooperation with departments of ophthalmology, audiology and
clinical genetics are essential.

Since some patients such as the elderly and the multihandicapped tolerate travelling poorly, the low-vision service will
profit from being part-time mobile, a bus can be converted
to meet this need.

References

Brinck HP, Aaved H, Eriksen HL, Sørheim H (1981) Øyebussen.
Ambulant øyelegetjeneste for distrikterne. Tidskr
Nor Lægeforen lol (29)163o-31.

Goldstein H.: Incidence, Prevalence and Causes of Blindness.
Publ. Health Rev. Vol. III, No. 1, 1974.

Henkind P, Suarez MF (1974) An urban eye clinic. The Sight-
Saving Rev. 44, 23-30.

Warburg M, Frederiksen P, Rattleff J (1979) Blindness among
77oo mentally retarded children. In: Smith V Keen
J (Eds) Visual handicap in children. Clinics in
Developmental Medicine No. 73. Spastics International
Med Publ. with Heinemann Med. London Philadelphia
pp 56-69.

Woodruff ME, Cleary TE, Bader D (1980) The prevalence of
refractive and ocular anomalies among 1242
institutionalized mentally retarded persons. Am.
J. Optometry Psys. optics 57:70-84.

READING BY THE ELDERLY (READING BY SUBJECTS WITH NORMAL AND LOW VISION)

D.H.A. Aberson
Institute for Perception Research
P.O.Box 513 - 5600 MB Eindhoven, Netherlands

1. INTRODUCTION

The printed word has become one of the most important means of acquiring information and of being able to carry out one's private affairs. In our society, therefore, people who have reading problems are severely handicapped. They have to cope with problems of isolation and dependence on other people. A large percentage of the population is visually handicapped. This percentage increases with age from less than 10% for people below 75 to 30% for people over 75 (Pitts, 1982). The main factors involved in loss of visual acuity associated with the aging process are retinal defects, decrease of accommodation capacity and transparency of the eye media, and excessive production of tears. Among people over 65, cataracts and glaucoma are roughly eight times more commom than in the general population and retinal disorders are six times more common. Roughly 5% of persons over 65 have visual impairments severe enough to prevent them from reading newspaper print with corrective spectacles (Greenberg & Branch, 1982). The older retina is said to receive only about one-third as much light as does its younger counterpart because of a smaller pupil size and changes in the optical media (Weale, 1961). The rate of recovery from glare is found to be significantly delayed in older persons (Reading, 1968). Age also produces decrements in visual field size, visual search performance and contrast sensitivity (Carter, 1982, Pitts, 1982). In most cases, however people retain some residual vision. The aged can usually continue to read ordinary text provided optimal conditions are created. This has some important advantages over braille. Firstly, when people become poorly sighted in old age it is difficult for them to master braille. Secondly, they can still deal with ordinary print on forms, advertisements, letters and newspapers, which keeps them more integrated in society. In addition, when such optimal conditions are created, people can also do their needlework or look at pictures and photographs.

Automatic speech production from visual displays provides no alternative solution, because the current form of man-machine dialogue is designed for visual presentation to the normally sighted and is not directly suitable for auditory presentation.

The aging process is known to bring about changes in behaviour and to affect functions other than purely visual ones which might be relevant to reading performance. Coates & Kirby (1982) and Salthouse (1982) mention an overall slowing of behavior, an increased variability between individuals when they become older. Welford (1958) observed that speed of reponse declines due to the extra time needed for initiation of the intended movement. Intelligence, memory and learning capacity as well as physical strength also show age related declines. Although much literature is available on these topics, not much is known about the influence of these factors on reading. During the last decade research into normal reading processes has been done at the Institute for Perception Research (Bouma, 1973, Bouma & de Voogd, 1974, Bouwhuis & Bouma, 1979). Our purpose is now to extend this fundamental knowledge with results from our present experiments on the reading processes of elderly (visually handicapped) people.

Furthermore, little is known about the effectiveness of various existing aids, other than spectacles, with respect to reading performance. Preliminary research has shown that character size, contrast and reading posture are relevant variables in this respect (Gabriëls, 1981). Attention needs to be paid to the perceptual effects of optical magnification, illumination quality, intensity and glare, and to ergonomic solutions which suit the reading habits of the elderly and their physical requirements.

Therefore, in order to develop useful aids and to be able to give appropriate advice, we need to gain fundamental knowledge about the reading processes of the elderly.

Last but not least, the resulting aids need to be produced and made available to those who could benefit from them. There must therefore be information about their existence, and they need to be subsidised or priced within the user's budget and accompanied by appropriate advice and manuals on their use.

2. READING RESEARCH

2.1 Normal visual reading process

The normal visual reading process is assumed to consist of 4 basic
processes:
- optical imaging
- control of eye saccades
- foveal and parafoveal word recognition
- integration of information over saccades

The actual perceiving takes place during the eye fixation pauses. These
last approximately 200-400 msec. The amount seen during such a fixation
pause is called the functional reading span.

This is typically 18 character widths centred around the fixation point in
the visual field, over a wide range of print sizes according to Rayner
(1983). In contrast, Tinker (1963) found an optimum print size in relation
to reading speed within a normal range of letter sizes.

Our hypothesis is that reading speed is directly related both to the
functional reading span and to the magnitude and frequency of saccades
between fixations. Our research programme therefore attempts to determine
important factors in these two processes for readers with normal and low
vision.

2.2 Experiments

In order to explore the visual reading processes of elderly people with
either normal or poor eyesight a series of experiments have been carried
out.

Firstly an experiment on reading aloud was performed with 47 subjects aged
from 35 to 75[+] with normal and low vision and an IQ above 100, together
with a control experiment on word recognition. The subjects were presented
with 10 texts of 5 different character heights ranging from

1.8. to 16 mm* and 3 levels of illumination ranging from 40 to 4000 lux.
Elderly subjects (65-75[+]) were found to have a slightly lower reading
speed than a control group (35-45) when reading aloud, though there was
considerable variance within and overlap between the scores for the two
groups. A ceiling effect was found for oral reading speed when reading
speed approached the subject's normal speaking rate.
The differences between the various age groups were suprisingly small. As
can be seen the difference between the high and low acuity subjects was
considerably greater for the younger than for the older readers.
All subjects appear to benefit slightly from the use of larger
letter, while those with poor visual acuity benefit to a relatively
greater extent. Reading speed is optimal with an intermediate
illumination level of 400 lux for people with both normal and low vision,
though the differences were small (see table I).

	40	400	4000	lux
NV	172	182	176	
LV	132	144	137	

Table I: Average reading speeds in words per minute for subjects with
normal and low vision for 3 levels of illuminance.

Subjects with normal vision do not like the extreme conditions with 9 and
16mm letters and an illumination level of 4000 lux, although their oral
reading speed is at its ceiling value under these conditions.
Even when subjects with low vision read under optimal conditions, they
do not equal the reading speed of subjects with normal vision.

* letters of 1.8-16mm lower case h height

In a word recognition experiment the same subjects were tachistoscopically
presented with 6-letter words, located foveally and parafoveally to the
right and left in the visual field (4 character widths from the center of
the visual field). Exposure duration was 100 msec (too short to change eye
fixation). Correct recognition scores and vocal reaction times were taken
as dependent variables.
As in the previous experiment, the illumination effects were marginal.
Figure 2 shows percentage correct as a function of letter size and visual
field position.

As expected, recognition scores are highest for foveal presentation,
followed by parafoveally right presentation, followed by left
presentation.
Once again the differences between the 40-60 and 70-80 age groups were
small. However, a clear difference now emerges between the normal and low
acuity groups. With foveal presentation recognition by the low acuity
group improves with increasing letter size, approaching that of the normal
group for the largest letters. With peripheral presentation, past a
certain peak, performance falls off equally for normal and low acuity
subjects, suggesting that there are limitations on the processing of large
characters.
Reaction times were not affected by illumination or magnification
differences, though the reaction times for subjects with low vision were
somewhat longer than for those with normal vision.
Since reading speeds approached normal speaking rates for the subjects in
the first experiment, this may have imposed an upper ceiling on the data.

It was therefore decided to investigate silent reading in the next
experiment. 18 Elderly persons between 65 and 75 with normal vision and a
control group of 15 subjects between 35 and 45 who also had normal vision
participated in the first pilot study. All had an IQ above 100. They were
presented with 12 texts with 6 letter sizes between 1 and 9 mm lower case
x height. A homogeneous illumination level of 1600 lux was employed.

Figure 3 shows reading speed as a function of letter size for subjects of
varying acuity. An optimum letter size of 3.8mm was found for subjects
with an acuity around 1.0, shifting to smaller letters for the sharp
sighted.
There was an apparent difference between age groups, with an average
reading rate of 246 w.p.m. for the elderly and 303 w.p.m. for the
controls. However, examination of those subjects with an identical acuity
of 1.4 (5 elderly and 4 control) reveals no age difference (see figure 4).

An incidental observation was that the subjects in the control group
showed a much greater range of reading rates than the elderly. Subsequent
analysis revealed that this was because of the male subjects in the
control group.

Relatively low reading speeds were found for the extremes of character
size.
The paradoxical increase in reading speed with 9 mm letters was consistent
over subjects, though informal observation suggests that this might be at
the expense of understanding what has been read.

3. CONCLUSIONS

It would appear from these findings that the principal problems for
elderly readers lie in their diminished visual acuity and not in more
general cognitive deficits. Therefore first priority should be given to
development of good visual aids.

As text presented on visual displays comes to play a larger role in
society, it seems particularly important to consider the often relatively
trivial modifications to these displays (such as variable letter size and
spacing, and presentation rate) which may make them available to those
with low vision.

4. REFERENCES

Bouma, H. (1973) 'Visual interference in the parafoveal recognition of initial and final letters of words. Vision Research 13, 767-782.

Bouma, H., de Voogd, A.H. (1974) 'On the control of eye saccades in reading'. Vision Research 14, 273-284.

Bouma H., Legein, Ch.P., Mélotte, H.E.M., Zabel, L. (1982) 'Is large print easy to read? Oral reading rate and word recognition of elderly subjects'. IPO Annual Progress Report 17, 84-91.

Bouwhuis, D.G., Bouma, H. (1979) 'Visual word recognition of three letter words as derived from the recognition of the constituent letters'. Perception and Psychophysics 25, 12-22.

Carter, J.H. (1982) 'The effects of aging upon selected visual functions: color vision, glare sensitivity, field of vision and accomodation'. in ed. Sekuler, R., Kline, D., Dismukes, K. vol. 2, Modern Aging Research, Alan R.Liss, Inc., New York.

Coates, G.D., Kirby, R.H. (1982) 'Organismic factors and individual differences in human performance and productivity'. Human Performance and Productivity, ed. Alluisi, E.A. & Fleisman, E.A., Vol.3, Hillsdale, N.J.: Lawrence Erlbaum Associates.

Gabriëls, S. (1981), IPO rapport no. 414

Greenberg, D.A. & Branch, L.G. (1982) 'A review of methodological issues concerning incidence and prevalence data of visual deterioration in elders'. in ed. Sekuler, R., Kline, D., Dismukes, K. vol. 2, Modern Aging Research, Alan R.Liss, Inc., New York.

Legein, Ch.P., Bouma, H. (1982) 'Reading and the ophtalmologist; an introduction into the complex phenomenon of ordinary reading as a guidance for analysis and treatment of disabled readers'. Documenta ophtalmologica, 53, 123-157.

Rayner, K. (1978) 'Eye movement in reading and information processing'. Psychological Bulletin, Vol. 85, no. 3, 618-660.

Reading, V. (1968) 'Disability glare & age vision' Res 8: 207-214.

Salthouse, T.A. (1982) 'Adult cognition'. New York, Springer.

Salthouse, T.A., Ellis, C.L. 'Determinants of eye fixation duration'. American Journal of Psychology. Vol.93, no.2, pp. 207-324, 1980.

Schiepers, C.W.J. (1980) Perception and Psychophysics 27, 71.

Silver, J.H. (1977) 'Low vision aids in the management of visual handicap'. Moorfields Eye Hospital, London.

Tinker, M.A. (1958) 'Recent studies of eye movements in reading'. Psychological Bulletin, 55, 215-231,

Weale, R.A. (1961) 'Retinal illumination and age'. Transaction of the Illumination Engineering Society, vol.26 no.2.

Welford, (1958) Aging and human skill, Oxford Press.

Zabel, L. (1983) IPO Rapport 426, Lezen bij Ouderen I.

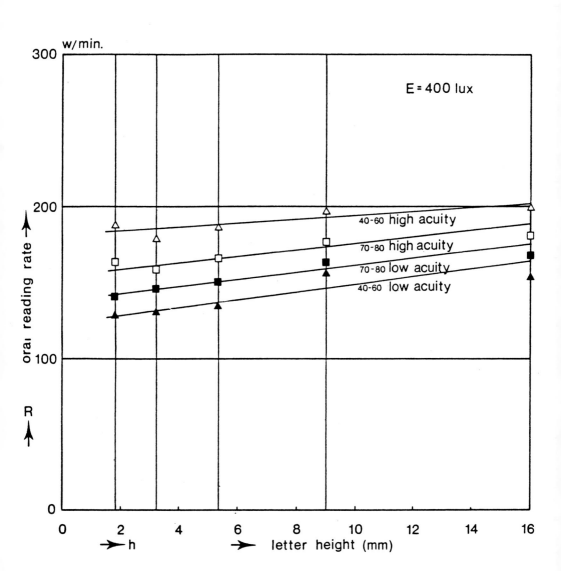

FIGURE 1

188

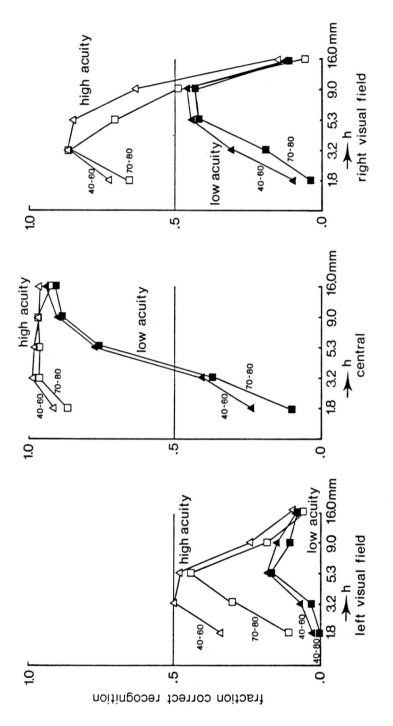

FIGURE 2

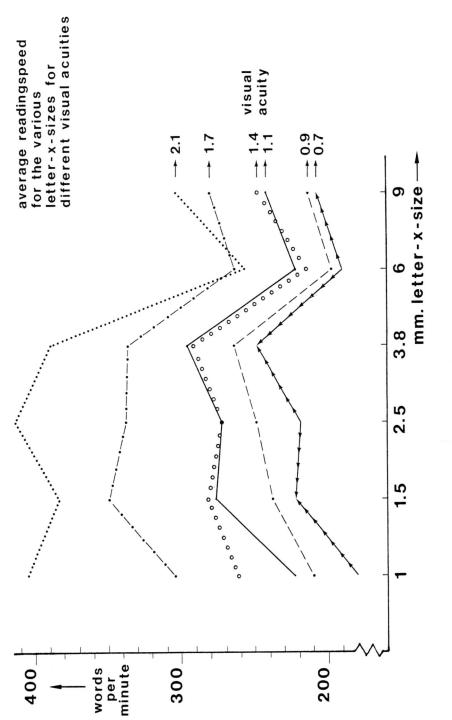

FIGURE 3

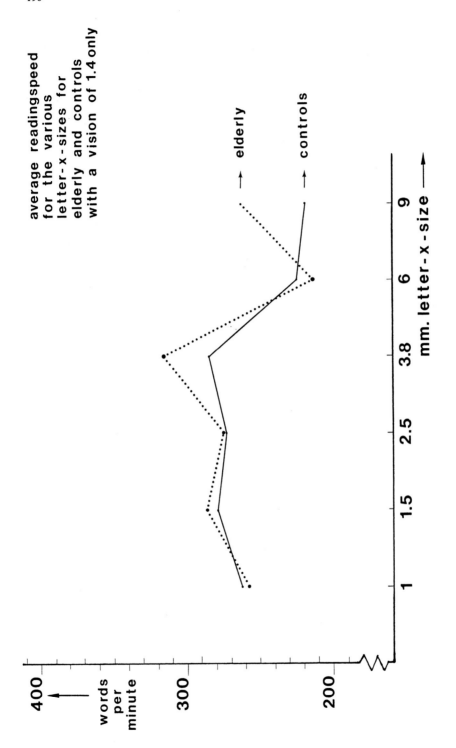

average readingspeed
for the various
letter-x-sizes for
elderly and controls
with a vision of 1.4 only

→ elderly

→ controls

FIGURE 4

ASSESSMENT OF THE NEEDS OF LOW-VISION PATIENTS

J.H. Silver
Moorfields Eye Hospital
City Road, London EC1V 2PD

WHO ARE THE BLIND ?

The classic image of a blind person is someone who has no perception of light is young, male, highly intelligent, with acute hearing and sensitivity. He has no other disabilities, is well equipped with sophisticated aids such as Sonic spectacles, has a guide dog and earns his living as a television detective or pop star. His blindness is either congenital or has been caused by some dramatic, usually traumatic event. His eyes have a normal appearance. This romantic image is a long way from reality, even in advanced countries. The visually handicapped person is most likely to have some useful vision, be female, elderly, unable to handle high technology aids even if they were available to her, and have one of the degenerative disorders which has been insidious rather than dramatic in onset. She no longer has paid employment, is keen to maintain her independence and may not be recognised by the community as having a disability at all (Cullinan 1977). Indeed one of the problems that occurs whenever blindness is discussed, is that to the lay person, blindness means no perception of light; a condition that occurs in less than 5 per cent of all those recognised as having a visual disability (Sorsby 1972).

The problems are compounded by the many definitions that are available. A brief search through the literature demonstrates at least 65 alternatives in use (Nizetic 1975). In advanced countries definitions tend to be based on levels of visual acuity, sometimes with field loss taken into account. In the third world they may be based on estimates of ability to function as a sighted person. In either case the biggest single problem with the statistics is that they are generally acknowledged to be totally inadequate with much blindness being totally unrecognised by the professionals working in the field. If we look at the prevalence of blind registration in the community in England and Wales the most recent figures suggest that if you are under the age of 65 you have one chance in a thousand (1.117/1000). If you are over 75 the rate is nearly 25/1000 (23.24/1000). Even more dramatically you are nearly 100 times more likely to be recognised as blind if you are over 75 then if you are under 16 years of age (DHSS 1983). The older you are the more likely you are to be female if you have a visual disability. The problem is likely to increase considerably by the end of the century (HMSO 1982).

HOW THE BLIND SEE

Generally speaking visual defects can be classified into main groups.

1. - Central Scotoma is by far the most significant group numerically. A central scotoma leaves mobility more or less unimpaired but prevents the individual from seeing up detail. Common causes are macular degeneration, optic atrophy, diabetic maculopathy, central serous retinopathy etc. This group are, without exception, unable to read small print with normal spectacles and also complain of difficulty with tasks that involve perception of small detail at any distance.

2. - An overall depression of visual acuity. This group would include albinism, certain corneal and vitreous disorders, monocular amblyopia (where the better eye has failed) etc.

3. - Where the light path is interrupted by scarring of the cornea, cataract, vitreous haemorrhage etc. This group tends to have fairly variable acuities, lots of problems with light scatter but need high levels of illumination and excellent contrast.

4. - Field Loss. This is another fairly variable group that may vary from the tunnel vision effects that are found at a late stage of classic retinitis pigmentosa or glaucoma to the hemianopias associated with neurological damage, or detached retinas etc. The disability will obviously depend upon the nature and position of the field loss.

AGE DISTRIBUTION

It is necessary further to divide the visual handicapped population into age groups. Here we must consider three main sub-divisions.

Under five year olds

Nearly all have a congenital disability and some 30% are likely to have at least one other disability too (Sorsby 1976). While numerically a very small number they are, of course, the most demanding in terms of patient years. They are the group for whom high technology aids are likely to be of great benefit in the future and who have sufficient flexibility to learn how to use them. Very often aids will need to be created specifically to individual needs if the childs abilities are to be stretched and he is to reach his full potential. Relatively few have the modality of sight totally absent and therefore need sight replacement techniques. Commonest causes of visual disability in this group are optic atrophy and congenital cataract, both of which allow the child some residual vision and enable him to get around using sighted methods. His greatest need is likely to be aids that will give him access to ink print.

Children.
Young people in education present a whole load of problems in terms of their place in the community, but if they are to be integrated which is the current social tendency, instruments that give them access to normal reading materials become a very high priority. Again relatively few are totally blind. Diagnostic groups are similar to group one but here conditions such as albinism have a significant impact.

It is important for the non-clinician to understand that different diagnoses give different perceptions of the world and the blind, apart from the few who are totally blind, are a widely disparate group with intelligence, dexterity and other personal qualities, such as persistence all modifying or alleviating the effect of the visual disability. In this second group the pigmentary degenerations become significant to as do retinal detachments etc.

Adults.
The third group, that is the people in the employable age group, present perhaps the biggest challenge. The largest single diagnostic group in this category is diabetic retinopathy. These patients present a range of problems. They have reduced sense of touch due to peripheral neuropathy and, therefore, do not do well with braille or similar media. Typically a diabetic will have acquired his disability at a time of peak responsibility, in his 30's or 40's, and his major need will be to sustain his previous activities despite his disability. Other major causes of blindness in this group are retinal detachments, myopia, uveitis, retinitis pigmentosa and the degenerative disorders start to become significant.

The Elderly.
In the fourth group by far the largest diagnosis is macular degeneration which is responsible, depending upon which authority is quoted, for anything up to one third of all recognised visual disabiltiy. Cataracts provide a very large sector of the aged visually handicapped population, the solution is, of course a surgical one, but there is often a waiting period, during which time there is a deficit that demands assistance. Elderly patients often find it very difficult to adapt to the use of other modalities and can unless given the appropriate assistance become a very considerable responsibility both to the community and individual responsible for their welfare. There major need is for aids that help them maintain their independence.

The advent of the intra-ocular lens has vastly improved the adaptation to aphakia which had been such a problem until recent years but the prevalence of other disabilites becomes

significant again in this age group with impaired grip, tremor
as well as poor motivation being very significant.

LOW VISION ASSESSMENT

In order to provide optimum aids for the low vision patient
the practitioner needs to have coherent, sensitive approach.
There is always the tendency to try to persuade people to do
what the Practitioner believes they should want to do, rather
than actually to solve the problems that the patient perceives
himself.

Low vision assessment is performed by different disciplines
in different places and in some countries it may be done by
teachers, social workers or other people with very little
knowledge of either ophthalmology or optics. For the purposes
of this paper it is assumed that the Practitioner has a
fundamental knowledge of Ophthalmology and a good knowledge of
optics, ie, is an Ophthalmologist or Optometrist. The most
important part of the low vision examination is to define the
tasks that the patient wishes to perform. It is common to be
presented with a very diffuse series of problems which amount
to 'I would really like to be able to see in the way that
people with normal eyes do' and it is has to be understood
clearly by the patient that no aids can replace lost sight and
every aid has disadvantages. The major function of the low
vision Practitioner is to solve as many problems as possible
while creating a few new ones. Most people will state a
primary need to read.This particulary applies to elderly
people where the loss of privacy involved in being unable to
manage day to day correspondence, read the instructions on
food packets and appliances and perhaps most importantly
medication can lead to a crucial loss of confidence and
dependence upon other people. Old people particularly if
recognised as 'blind° will have low expectations, the young
will feel themselves to be stigmatised and isolated. It is not
enough to know that someone wishes to be able to read. It is
important to know whether the reading is the odd day-to-day
letter or hours of concentrated study making notes at the same
time, whether the notes are made by hand, type-script, tape
recorder and so on.

When subjects are in the employable age groups assessment
demands not only an analysis of the present task, but since
many visually handicapped people are functioning at well below
their optimum level an investigation of the patients potential
talents and abilities. Discussion will elicit much useful
information about the career possibilities of any individual.

If the problems stated are for distance vision, it is
necessary to understand whether they are general mobility or a
specific need to see perhaps a blackboard, a bus number or
even a bus. The Practitioner will need to know how the
patient perceives the world. The type of visual disability

and to some extent the prognosis has a bearing on the prescribing philosophy.

Any basic refractive error must be corrected, and the best level of reading acuity established with a normal spectacle correction. Levels of optical magnification are established for each eye separately and the possibility of binocular function investigated. If the tasks have been analysed properly then the most appropriate type of aid is clearly indicated and in the first instance the patient's response to this should be assessed. It is also sound practice to demonstrate aids of alternative types partly because they often elicit other problems that may not have been voiced in the preliminary discussions, and partly because the optimum aid may not be acceptable to the patient and this may cause him to revise his original requests.
It is in the work environment that microprocessors allied to sophisticated aids have their greatest possibilities. Low vision assessment must be modified if CCTV is being considered. Certain diagnostic groups seem to be able to use sight with CCTV when the same level of optical magnification is inadequate. Notable here are retinitis pigmentosa, where apparently a picture is built up by some sort of scanning strategy. Disorders where very high contrast levels are needed such as anterior uveitis and the corneal dystrophies also benefit from reversed contrast (i.e white print on a black background) and the reduction of glare so produced. There is evidence that a black on white image is generally preferable (Mehr et al 1977), but of course the alternative option is necessary for pictures etc. Magnification can be recorded by the use of two rulers, once the optimum magnification for the task is established, one ruler is shown on the screen, the other measures one unit on it. The viewing distance is recorded aswell, and the patient must be wearing the appropriate optical correction.

WHERE THE NEW TECHNOLOGY CAN HELP

There exists a considerable demand for a portable electronic aid which has the characteristics, in particular the flexibilty of CCTV. It is possible to envisage a flat screen with a camera on a sort of cantilevered arm that swings out of case comparable to a brief case.

While the vast majority of low vision patients are elderly and do have marked resistence to complex high technology aids; it would seem that the intelligent application of microprocessors should be able to simplfy some of their day to day living problems. Optical into sound systems must have a place in this. For example a system that will enable an elderly person to admit to her home automatically a list of recognisable individuals could be an advantage.

Clearly microprocessors are likely to be of use to extend the range of available aids. Machines that will read print aloud are already available but financially quite beyond the reach of the average private individual who is often, by the nature of her disability, unable to go to an institution such as a public library where such machines might be available. An optical recognition system that would be able to interpret hand writing is clearly needed as is an inexpensive way of tranferring the spoken word, that is an audible signal, into ink print or braille. Devices that respond to verbal signals already exist,a machine that will type a dictated letter must be possible, and while obviously prohibitively expensive on an individual basis, the use of a telephone link to a computer system seems feasible.

A device that automatically recognises the right bus and stops it would have a place.

The next generation of electronic aids will need to be more flexible and adapt to the vary needs of individual patients perhaps on a modular basis.

N.B. In this paper all examples and statistics have been taken from the U.K. sources. There is no reason to believe that there are any significant differences between the European countries or North America.

REFERENCES

Cullinan,T.R.(1977) Visually disabled people in the community. Health Services Research Unit Report 28. University of Kent at Canterbury.
Department of Health and Social Security.(1983) Registered blind and partially sighted persons. Year ending March 31st 1981
HMSO (1982) Population Projections to 1990. HMSO
Mehr,E.B.,Frost,A.B., and Apple,L.E.(1977) Experience with Closed circuit television in the Blind Veterans Administration. Am.J. Optom 50, 6 458-469.
Nizetic,B. (1975) Public Health Ophthalmology. Theory and Practice of Public Health. Editor W.Hobson Oxford Medical Publications.
Sorsby, A.(1972) The incidence and causes of blindness in England and Wales 1963-1968. DHSS Reports on Health and Medical Subjects No 128 DHSS London.

LOW VISION AIDS AND SOME PERCEPTUAL ASPECTS OF READING BY THE PARTIALLY SIGHTED

M.J. Tobin
Research Centre for the Education of the Visually Handicapped
University of Birmingham
Selly Wick House, 59 Selly Wick Road, Birmingham, B29 7JE, England

Before the specific problems hinted at by the title of this presentation are directly addressed, it may be useful to remind ourselves that partially sighted people are not a homogeneous group, with a readily discernible set of reading difficulties. Not only are they as variable as the whole population of human beings in terms of general health, intelligence, social/economic background, motivation, etc., they are also different from one another in terms of the causation of their visual impairment and of their measured visual acuities. Unlike the totally blind or those with light-perception — for whom no printed text is of any direct value whatsoever — the partially sighted can be helped to decode print in a variety of ways. Magnification of the print stimuli (by means of spectacles, hand-held or hand-operated low-vision aids, or by bringing the text closer to the eye) is one familiar procedure. Enhancement of the image by altering the colour of, and/or the contrast between, the 'figure' and its background is another effective method for some of them. However, merely knowing what the cause of the impairment may be, or knowing what the objectively-measured acuities are recorded as, will tell us very little about how effective a reader a given person will be. As a group of 'patients', or 'clients', they will not, even within such a narrowly de-limited activity as the reading of print text, present themselves as having similar problems, similar strategies for overcoming those problems, and with comparable levels of achievement. In stating what is no doubt obvious to us all, it is my intention to underline the fact that the design of physical devices (a) must be informed by a lively awareness of the individual differences among this group of fellow human-beings and (b) must ensure that there is a 'built-in' flexibility, a 'built-in' facility for total control by the users themselves.

When the psychologist or educationalist talks about perceptual factors in relation to reading, he is usually thinking of such activities as pattern matching and discrimination, letter reversals and inversions and transpositions, the sequential analysis/registration of letters within words, and the left-to-right 'scanning' of words and phrases within sentences. The kind of research that may guide and direct the work of the perceptual psychologist who turns his attention for a moment to the problems associated with the de-coding of print would be, just to cite one example, that which has found there to be a 'centre-outwards' scanning strategy for strings of two-dimensional shapes among adults but a left-to-right scanning strategy for strings of letters (Figure 1). This left-to-right scanning procedure seems on the surface to be optimal for en-coding letter-order in Western (as opposed of course to Arabic or Hebraic) script, and it may be highly 'adaptive', to use some of the psychological jargon, in word recognition. This would constitute an important sub-skill in reading development, and failure to master it would lead an educational psychologist or perceptual psychologist to predict lower levels of reading accuracy and lower levels of reading speed among children who were still relying too heavily on the 'centre-out' scanning procedure. The psychologist would not want to claim too much for the left-to-right strategy, however, and indeed in very long words, such as the English 'A N T I D I S E S T A B L I S H M E N T A R I A N I S M' (Figure 1), a mixture of left-to-right, centre-out, and even right-to-left modes of attack may have to be invoked for quick and successful de-coding. What this illustrates, perhaps, is that the skilful adult reader has a <u>set</u> of scanning strategies available for use in what Goodman (1967) has labelled as the 'psycholinguistic guessing game', viz. the act of reading. Among its implications for the designers of devices, lenses, image-enhancers, etc., one of the most important is that in magnifying the physical stimulus beyond a certain level they may be creating an entirely new set of difficulties for the reader. In improving the quality of the image falling upon the retina, they may indeed be precluding the rapid invoking of alternative scanning strategies; in improving one aspect of the perception of the stimulus, they may be spoiling another. Moreover, they may be generating an entirely different problem, different in the sense that it has a greater cognitive loading as opposed to a perceptual loading.

FIGURE 1.

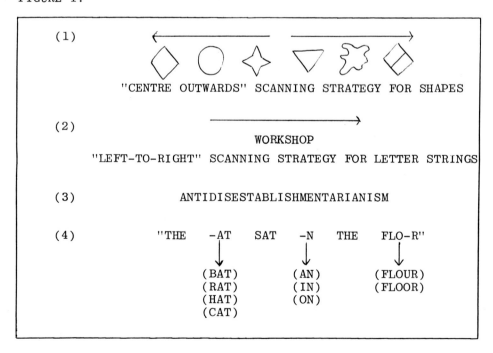

Goodman's phrase, 'psycholinguistic guessing game', is apposite
again at this point. On the one hand it reminds us that reading is possible without our having to 'perceive' every letter
or even every word. As children, our growing knowledge about
the structure of our native language — about its syntactic
and semantic regularities for example — allows us to guess
what has been accidentally omitted and to predict what should
follow with a very high degree of precision. If we look at
the sentence "THE -AT SAT -N THE FLO-R", we all know enough
about the grammatical rules that operate in English to guess
what it probably should be. In other words, cognitive factors
also operate in our de-coding of text and may be able to
compensate for deficiencies in visual perception, whether those
deficiencies are attributable to the poor quality of the external, physical stimulus or to the impairment of the ocular
apparatus as in such conditions as albinism or nystagmus.
Goodman's description is useful in another way in pointing up
the cognitive component in reading. It implies the operation
of memory, and not only the 'long-term' memory that mediates
our use of the grammatical rules and the probabilities of
occurrence of specific letters, groups of letters, and words.
It is that other kind of memory that is being considered at the
moment, the one that psychologists call 'short-term' memory.
It is the memory capacity we use when asking someone for a
telephone number that we intend to dial immediately, and then
forget because it will no longer be of use to us and will not,
therefore, be passed on for retention in the long-term store.
It is the memory capacity we use when reading a sentence. We
have to hold in temporary storage the words we have just perceived until we have enough information available to extract
the full meaning of the sentence. Having done that, we can
then jettison, forget, the earlier words completely. But
enough of them have to be retained in what is a limited space
until we can 'close in' on the intended, or inferred, meaning.
The inventor of an aid that enhances perception of letters or
small groups of letters, and by doing so reduces the size of
the visual field to a very few letters, may indeed have improved
perception of small parts of what has to be de-coded, but he may
be doing it at the expense of cognition, especially that part of
cognition we call memory. One problem is solved by creating a
new one! And is the reader better off or worse off? This can
be left for our discussion session.

It may now be opportune to look at the results of a small part
of a longitudinal investigation that we have been conducting
with a group of blind and partially sighted children over the
past ten years. The enquiry is trying to plot the course of
intellectual development and school achievement in a cohort of
children who were aged five years in 1973 and who are now aged
15. We have tested them on a variety of measures over that
period but for our present discussion, attention is directed
solely on progress in reading, and specifically on speed of
reading as assessed with the Neale Analysis of Reading Ability
Test.

Using the norms from the normally-sighted population on which
the test was standardized, we observed, first of all, that as
the mean chronological age of the group increased from seven

years eight months to ten years seven months to eleven years
ten months, there was also an increase in their mean speed/rate
of reading, expressed here in terms of 'reading age'. We
observed also that the disparity between mean chronological
age and mean reading-speed age increased from each testing to
the next. At seven years eight months, they were measured as
being two months behind their normally-sighted peers; at ten
years seven months, they were thirty months behind; and at
eleven years ten months, they were thirty-seven months behind.

To demonstrate that it is not merely a case of this group being
atypical, unrepresentative, of the low vision population, an
entirely different group of children of different ages was also
tested. Although the details are different, the pattern is the
same — an ever-growing disparity between the partially sighted
and the normally sighted in the speed at which they can process
visually-presented material. Again, interpretation and
explanation' can be left to our discussion session.

To conclude, I would wish to suggest that the designers of low-
vision aids should examine the empirical data on perception and
about achievement, and ask themselves whether they are giving
due attention to the important perceptual and cognitive aspects
of the problem. Does, for example, their new invention allow
alternative scanning strategies or procedures to be invoked by
the reader at will? Does it so restrict the width and depth of
the visual 'window' or field, that the reader can no longer
make use of the information provided by indenting, paragraphing,
underlining, italicizing, etc? Does the device require such
delicate psycho-motor manipulation skills that it is of reduced
value to young children, to the elderly, and to the additionally
handicapped? Does it permit image inversion (white on black),
variation in brightness of figure and ground, and level of
contrast between them? Does it produce a wavering, unstable
image that will exacerbate the difficulties of those who suffer
from nystagmus? Can the plane of the stimulus, the image, be
altered between the horizontal and the vertical? Is it just
a reading device or can it be used when the operator wants to
monitor his own writing? Is it portable? Is it cheap? Does
it entail a long training period by the user?

What, finally, are the criteria, the desirable standards, that
should be aimed at? Can they be determined in relation to
specific sub-groups so that proper attention — within reasonable engineering and commercial limits — can be paid to
individual differences among the users? A paper, then, that
asks more than it answers — but perhaps that is not inappropriate in a 'workshop'.

REFERENCES

GOODMAN, K.S. (1967). "Reading: a psycholinguistic guessing
game." Journal of the Reading Specialist, 6, 126-135.

VISUAL IMPAIRMENT IN GREECE: HEALTH SERVICE ORGANIZATION

J. Levett, Athens School of Public Health
J. Yfantopoulos, Ministry of Health and Welfare
J. Tsamparlakis, Ophthalmiatrion Eye Hospital

INTRODUCTION

Disability related to sensory impairment is a relatively neglected health care problem in Greece today.While the problem is
likely to grow in severity,rehabilitation service policy making is marginally integrated into overall health care and
sensory impairment services are undeveloped in the European
context.Bearing in mind that sensory impairment and related
disabilities constitute a set of prevalent afflictions globally and that a systematic approach has been partially developed
in Europe,the Greek problem by comparison demands serious attention .

A HISTORICAL EVOLUTION OF THE EYE CARE IN GREECE

After the establishment of a modern Greek State,various ethnic,
political,economic and social forces have influenced and shaped
the development of medical services.
The greatest challenge of ophthalmology was the control and
eradication of infectious diseases of the external membranes,
mainly trachoma which until the 1930 s was the leading cause
of blindness.The main ophthalmological center in Greece until
the 1950 s was the "Ophthalmiatrion",housing the University
Clinic and linked to important eye-centers in continental Europe.
Subsequent to the second world war,young ophthalmologists were
attracted more to both British and American centers especially
for postgraduate training and clinical research.
Today Greece has four active university eye centers and an
adequate number of ophthalmologists.Clinical diagnosis and
therapy present no particular problem and complicated surgery
is undertaken routinely.Post-operative care,follow-up and technological support represent some of the local problems.

202

EPIDEMIOLOGICAL ASPECTS OF VISUAL IMPAIRMENT

In Greece there are various sources of information on blindness.
However reported statistics are characterized by variability
and in some cases there is an underreporting of the real situation.
The official census of blind persons is obtained from lists,
kept in various registries.
It shows a registration of 11,615 (6080 male/5535 female)for
1960, 13.198 in 1970 and more than 14.000 in 1980.The age distribution of blind people in Greece is skewed towards the elderly and the young with the highest proportion in the aged
population (figure 1).Today there are few surviving persons
with trachoma and no clinically important new cases of chla-
mydia infections.Herpes simplex keratoconjuctivitis of the outer eye is the only present blinding infectious disease.It af-
fects seriously only a small number of individuals (figure 2).
The epidemiological pattern of visual impairment is converging
to that seen in other Western European countries with the main
cause of visual impairment being diabetes vasculopathies,glau-
coma,industrial and motor vehicle accidents,senile macular degeneration,genetically determined disease and the syndrome of
prematurity.Both rehabilitation and "continuity of care" of the
visually handicapped constitute one of the greatest challenges
to ophthalmology today.Traditional beliefs and societal attitudes towards blindness,visual disability and the attitudes of
the victim himself,constitute major obstacles towards improvement in early detection,effectiveness of care and rehabilitation. Ophthalmology has given insufficient emphasis to a suitable low-vision rehabilitation model for Greece and the movement for popular education has paid little heed to the overall
health care problem.
Health policies are only embryonically developed in the direction of promotion and protection of eye health.Financial resources available for low vision are considered inadequate.
According to the ophthalmological literature numerous definitions of visual disability exist.
This creates problems in standardization,classification and
comparison even within a single nation.According to one study,

less than 5% of the population designated as visually disabled,
demonstrated true blindness or a total absence of light perce-
ption.Therefore,complete and accurate descriptions of visual
disability are frequently lacking.Visual acuity with or without visual field mapping is reported in the developed na-
tions.In the developing nations,visual disability assessment
is frequently defined in terms of loss of normal functional
ability.Greece can be placed somewhere,in between these two
worlds in that visual impairment data is often comprehensive in
ophthalmological centers and not always complete in centrally
reported data.Discrepancies or contradictions can also be found
between original sources and reported estimates.However the
discovery of a serious visual impairment carries with it a high
probability that the individual will be defined as legally
blind.This "bias" results in the neglected use of all residual
vision in a significant portion of the visually impaired population.

PROVISION OF EYE CARE SERVICES IN GREECE:

Legislation:

In 1951 the first law (Law 1904) on prevention and rehabilitation of the blind was passed.It provided for the establishment
of a special body under the chairmanship of the General Secretary of the Ministry of Health for the prevention of blindness.
In 1952 a Royal decree was enacted that permitted blind children to be enrolled in regular schools and in 1956 a school
for blind telephone operators was established.In 1975 Law 37
was passed and according to Article 2,blind persons can register for courses of higher education.In 1979,Law 988 defined
legal blindness as 1/20.

Hospital Beds.

In 1981 there were 231 ophthalmological beds in Greek hospitals or 2.4 beds per 100.000 inhabitants.(Table 1).The regional distribution of ophthalmological beds is uneven.
Certain regions (Epirus,Thrace,Ionian and Aegean Islands) lack

204

a single bed.Other regions (Crete and Thessaly) have relatively
high bed rates (9.6 beds/100.000 population and 7.9/100.000 respectively).The recent establishment (1983) of a National
Health Service in Greece carries with it the expectation of a
reallocation of a ophthalmological resources.

Manpower.

The total number of ophthalmologists in Greece is 725 (or 7.25/
100.000 inhabitants). More than 50% of the total number of ophthalmologists are concentrated in the Athens area (Table 1)
where the 31% of the Greek population live.The rest are rather
evenly distributed throughout the regions.An adequate number
of ophthalmologists are found in regions lacking ophthalmological beds.

Technological Advances.

Advances in medical technology,applicable to rehabilitation of
the disabled have penetrated the Greek health care scene,not
however in a systematic and regulated fashion. Rehabilitation
engineering and biomedical engineering training programmes in
either university or medical school settings are non existent.
Medical technology assessment is sporadic and monpower needs
for its maintenance and routine inspection is inadequate.Where
present it is incompletely trained.Not a single highly trained
senior full time biomedical engineer is to be found in any Greek
hospital while major University teaching hospitals have not
established small groups of biomedical engineers.
Inadequacies in the availability of technological aids and
their poor distribution limit the access of children with visual
impairment to school reading material. A coordinated effort
could facilitate the application of microprocessorsand other a-
vailable and emerging technology in the service of rehabilita-
tion.A unique opportunity currently exists,through the emphasis on informatics recently placed by the Ministry of Research
and Technology.

Special Services and training programmes.

Special services and training programmes for the rehabilitation
of the disabled vary in quality and far from meet existing national needs.Two schools exist for blind children as well as
an institution for the professional orientation of partially
sighted adolescents.Organized rehabilitation services do not
exist for adults and aged partially sighted or blind persons.
Rehabilitation health service policy making and policy makers
often lack a modern conceptual framework that would ensure both
the integration of comprehensive rehabilitation into the overall
health care system and the needed participation of adequate
numbers of behavioural scientists.Health service development
has been impeded by the proliferation of numerous models and
sub-models for health care coverage and its effective and accurate evaluation questioned or obstructed as a result of inadequate documentation and fuzzy data.Consequently,multidisiplina-
ry research activities in rehabilitation medicine and concomi-
tant health services are non-existent. In the absence of in-
centives the individual with the visual impairment is "directed"
and motivated by the availability of a subsidy or allowance for
the blind.Lack of job-incentives for the partially sighted reduce the interest in visual training and vocational rehabilitation.

PREVENTIVE AND WELFARE PROGRAMMES.

Prevention

In recent years various health prevention and health promotion
programmes have been established.
Directed mainly to the prevention of eye-disease in school children,they have developed in two stages.The first covers a school
check-up or screening by trained teachers.The second stage
covers futher eye and vision examinations undertaken by ophthalmologists.
In the period 1981-1982,170.000 school children underwent a stage 1 check-up.
Approximately 6000 children (3.6%) were found to have a visual

206

problem (<4/10) and were referred to stage 2.
3.800 (2.3%) children were given spectacles thereby improving
their vision to 10/10.The remainder underwent additional examination and some from of treatment was provided.

Allowances.

Welfare programmes for the blind are rather restricted.Never-
theless,various policies have been adopted to foster registration for the distribution of welfare benefits.According to a
recent census the number of eligible persons who can benefit
from an allowance is estimated to be 15.500.
Efforts made to ensure registration throughout Greece have resulted in a rather even regional participation (Table 1).
The social and welfare service consequently,is reasonably effective and by comparison more effective than the distribution
of medical services.

A MODEL FOR EYE-CARE

There is a growing awareness of the need for the application of
systems thinking and economic analysis to the rational development and evaluation of all aspects of Health Care Systems.In the
following analysis,a methodology is adopted to examine the Greek
Health Care Sector and to demonstrate qualitatively a comprehensive system of coverage.An idealized model for eye-care (health)
is presented (figure 3).Health care is seen as a staged process
over space and time. It contains the principle of "continuity
of care" either throughout life or throughout sickness and disease,individually and collectively.
Stage 1 of the Health Care System is the promotion or protection
of eye health and corresponds to preventive ophthalmology.Stage
2 is the early detection of visual problems necessitating targeted screening of high risk groups.To be effective appropriate
technologies most be utilised.Stage 3 and 4 cover diagnosis and
therapy,or traditional medicine,while stage 5 covers all aspects
of rehabilitation,representing physiatry or rehabilitation medicine.

Qualitatively from left to right,the severity of disease is
considered to be progressive from symptoms to impairment to
disability and the cumulative cost grows both individually
and collectively.The individual becomes less productive with
a dimminshed quality of life.To maintain life s quality,whi-
le minimizing the overall cost of care,prevention and early
detection of eye problems is stressed by the model.Education
of the population,especially children and the elderly is important to the effectiveness of steps 1 and 2.A low vision
facility,ideally houses a multidisiplinary team where persons
might be grouped into the partially sighted and the blind.
The rehabilitation programme is then adapted to each individuals unique profile.Consequently,through teamwork(educational,psychological sociological and medical) and the use of
suitable aids or appropriate medical technology,the individual
can be readapted to his environment cr the environment can be
"restructured" to the needs of the impaired individual.
Finally the visually impaired individual should be treated as
a "normal" person in that accessibility of services normally
available to all members of society should be available to him.
These might include Braille libraries for educational and re-
creational purposes,or communication facilities such as the
specially adapted telephone.It would also include auditory
signals at street crossings as a substitute for colour coded
"stop-go" information,or elevator information posted in Braille.
At the bottom of figure 3 a qualitative assessment,interpreted
either in terms of "priorities" or in terms of "outcome" is
provided.The current Greek model works well in the traditional
sense.Diagnosis and treatment of patients who find their way
into health care system is effective.It has suffered from neg-
lect in both prevention and rehabilitation with an unexpressed
demand or unmet need in the area of early detection,through
suitably targeted screeming strategies.Traditional medicine
(ophthalmology) receives a relatively high priority in that
the number of ophthalmologists is more than adequate to meet
the populations needs but they are poorly distributed.
In the absence of Familly doctors and suitable services the
patient has direct access to the specialist,a costly way in

general to provide service.Preventive ophthalomology has a low
but increasing priority and rehabilitation a non-priority.
The application of an evaluation model is therefore premature
though potentially useful in light of the new law for health
care and the development of a comprehensive national health
care system.An assessment of the Greek situation reveals the
need for accurate and more complete data collection to assess
age and population distribution of the visually impaired,the
cause of such impairments and the need for classification standards.
There is a need for Greece to implement a multidisiplinary low
vision facility whose function is the assessment of impairment,
implementation of corrective patient strategies and the directed training of patients,thus accomplishing the final stages
of our ideal model, or the overall rehabilitation of individuals with residual sight and those without.It is also important,that health care committees within the Ministry of Health are made more aware of manpower needs in the area of reha-
bilitation.The specialist professions themselves must also
stress the need for continuing education in their own specia-
lties and become more aware of the needed contributions of
other specialists such as psychologists,biomedical engineers
(man-machine systems) special counsellors or therapists.Socio-
logists for example are needed to assess the attitudes of visually impaired patients to their disability and the attitudes
of Greek society towards visual impairment.
The absence of educational programmes in biomedical engineering
covering aids technology and the man-machine interface or in
neurophysiology for research training into visual function,
or sensory substitution,impedes the local evaluation of aids
and prosthetics,the local development of screening technologies
for the assessment of visual performance in the real environment and science and technology transfer of research findings
into practical situations.

209

CONCLUSIONS

Visual handicap as in other nations is a problematic subject.
Greece lags behind other member nations of the EEC and all
northern European nations in low vision facility development,
basic clinical research in the visual sciences and in rehabilitation engineering.Rehabilitation of the visually impaired
has a low priority in the health care system,which is "biased"
towards a "waste" of residual visual function.Further more,
available services and health care coverage is less than adequate to meet the existing regional demand and unmet need e-
ven in a traditional sense.The infrastructure necessary to
the development of a comprehensive multidisiplinary low vision facility is lacking.The recently enacted law for the
establishment of a national health care system, while under-
scoring prevention and stating as its goal,free health care
for all according to need,relegates rehabilitation to a low
priority.The concept of continuity of care while implicit
in the new law,does not explicilty include rehabilitation
of the partially sighted or blind individual.To promote the
concept of continuity of eye care,certain priority areas must
be stressed and certain programmes implemented,as prerequi-
sities. These include the development of a scientific and technological base through the inauguration of post-graduate
training programmes in biomedical engineering and informatics,
special manpower considerations in the behavioural sciences,
systematic approachs to the organization and evaluation of
health care services and refinement of health care policy.

References

-Chapman,E.K.,Visually handicapped children, Routledge and
 Kegan,London 1978.
-Dimolitsa,A.,Legal and administrative measures for the blind,
 Athens 1980 (in Greek).
-Greek Statistical Services,Annual Reports.
-Kofinas,H.,Blindness in Greece,Arch.Hyg.,Athens 1975 (in
 Greek).

-Michaelson, I.C.,in Scientific foundations of ophthalmology
Ed.Perkins and Hill,William Heinemann Med.,1977.
-Nizetic,B.,in Theory and Practice of Public Health Ed.Hobson,
Oxford Medical,1975.
-WHO EURO Reports + Studies 41,The use of residual vision,1981.
-Yfantopoulos,J.,Economics of health status and health care
planning (Greece).D.Phil.,U.of York,1979.

TABLE 1

REGIONAL DISTRIBUTION OF THE EYE CARE SERVICES

REGION	ABSOLUTE NUMBERS					PER 100.000 POP.		
	DOCTORS	BEDS	IMPAIRED	POPULATION(10^6)	ALLOWANCES (10^6)	DOCTORS	BEDS	IMPAIRED
ATHENS	365	62	2,113	3,0	130.8	12.1	2.1	70.0
REST	360	169	13,360	6,7	673.6	5.4	2.5	199.7
GREECE	725	231	15,473	9,7	814.4	7.5	2.4	159.4

FIGURE 1

BLINDNESS IN GREECE ACCORDING TO AGE DISTRIBUTION

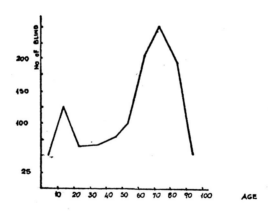

FIGURE 2.

DISEASE DISTRIBUTION IN PERCENTAGES

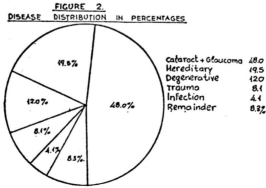

Cataract + Glaucoma 48.0
Hereditary 19.5
Degenerative 12.0
Trauma 8.1
Infection 4.1
Remainder 8.3%

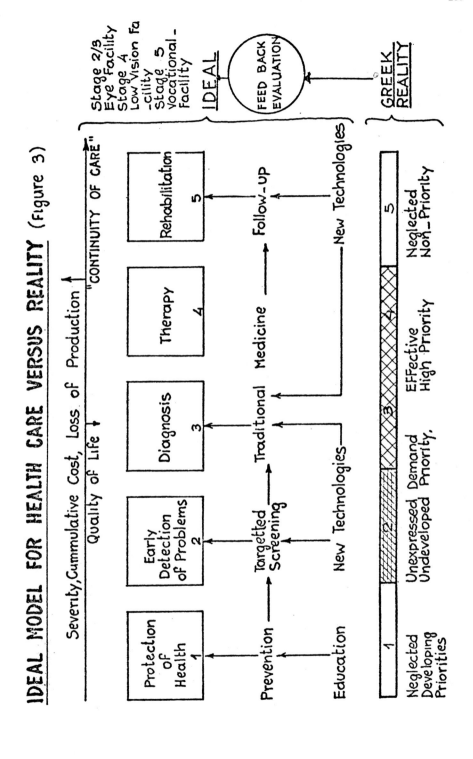

IDEAL MODEL FOR HEALTH CARE VERSUS REALITY (Figure 3)

NECESSITY OF AN INTERFACE BETWEEN RESEARCH OUTPUT AND SOCIAL NEEDS

M.I. Campo, A. Testa
Centro Socio Assistenziale "David Chiossone"
Unità Operativa del Consiglio Nazionale delle Ricerche
Progetto Finalizzato: Tecnologie Biomediche e Sanitarie
Corso Armellini, 11 - 16122 Genova

An overview of the literature dealing with all aspects of low vision can easily lead to a curious observation: first of all we can find medical and optical material; perceptual and cognitive investigations; technological research and descriptions of instruments and, last of all, teaching methodologies and rehabilitation tecniques. On the contrary it seems very difficult to find interdisciplinary approaches and cross reference information.

In fact this "no man's land" (as low vision is defined by E. Chapman (1)) is a wide and problematic area, where many different competences are needed and involved. Between blindness and sight we have a wide variety of types of pathologies and levels of efficiency. As a consequence many different points of view and/or lines of intervention may be applicable, each of them correct and just in itself but insufficient without the knowledge and the help of all the others.

This is true not only because of the wide range of subjects which go to make up the vague definition, but also for the difficulties deriving from the different languages spoken by the different specialists involved in the matter.

Ophthalmologists, opticians, neurologists, psychologists, biomedical engineers, rehabilitation workers, teachers, all have different (and often unknown to each other) theoretical assumptions, approaches and methodologies.

But, what is more important, often none of them are aware of the needs of their "customers".

This is what we have decided to call "social needs".

Actually they are needs of a particular society that is or should or tries to be integrated in the wider general society beginning from the family through the school, up to the vocational and professional world.

It is very common to find expert specialists in each of the cited disciplines, but it is very hard to find someone with the means to understand the general problems of this minority and give them specific counseling as regards combined clinical, pedagogical and technological aspects. This is not a presumption of encyclopedic knowledge but a call for an interdi-

sciplinary structure composed of professionals of different
expertise who can face together the various and often contradictory problems.
This is what we have called "interface between research output
and social needs".
The trend of this first workshop on rehabilitation of the visually impaired is to establish an European point of view
common to various competences: biomedical engineering first of
all, but also ophtalmology, pedagogy, psychology and rehabilitation methodologies in general.
Otherwise, it wouldn't be easy for a biomedical engineer to
develop a new aid without a feed back and an evalutation of
it by the users and, on their behalf, by the clinicians involved in this activity. It is important to achieve: identification of disabilities and related social needs; development of
training and methodologies for the use of the aids; rehabilita
tion programs; production and dissemination of the aids. The
absence of the users and the producers of these aids here today is therefore significant. With this evidence, my intention is not to make superficial criticism but to affirm future possibilities: this is a promotional workshop and it may
even be difficult for those present to understand each other
without introducing non specialists. Everyone can develop in
his own country the programs he believes to be most useful for
his purpose and consequently share his experience with all the
other countries.
In any case I can't see how we can work without the participa
tion of who profits from our research and specialization, and
of the producers of the aids.
This uninitiated but not alien presence, that of the social
needs expressed by this minority, could be of great help in
a correct interpretation and solution of our research output.
Now, since we cannot consider it possible to have direct con-
frontation with users and potential producers, we need an
"interface of multiple competences" between technological and
methodological research on one side, and social needs on the
other.
We need an intelligent and interdisciplinary filter which can
understand and interpret the actual needs of the users and
integrate them with the development and the level of research
in the field.
Let us see, in the absence of such a structure what is usually
the educational iter of a low vision patient in Italy, but, I
think, not only in our country (2): when low vision is disco-
vered, the patient is often defined as "legally blind" and,
as a consequence, educated as a blind person, thereby under-
using his residual vision and adopting Braille and other tecniques for totally blind.

Otherwise, he is classified as "sighted" and educated without
any special methodology. In this case, his residual vision is
often unused and ineffective. In both cases, it would be a
waste of time to emphasize the social and psychological conse
quences of the two kinds of curriculum. But in any case modern technologies and methodologies used to face the problems
of low vision are not taken into account.
It is a false problem if blind people should or should not use
technologies. Their and our aim should be to allow them to
live in the least restrict environment as possible and if
technologies serve to this purpose, welcome technologies and
their correct use.
It is obvious that the existence of a filter, leading to a wi
ser and more efficient use, to be made of the health organiza
tions as regards diagnosis and prognosis, able to know and
choose the appropriate technologies, elaborate the right methodologies and training; and finally guide the patient to pos
sible vocational activities, would be of great help.
This kind of center/structure involves the following fiels of
competence: experimentation, research, training of skilled per
sonnel, evalutation of technologies, vocational couseling.
We think that these aspects can constitute a good basis for
efficient rehabilitation methodologies.
Our center is trying to set up a structure of intervention
corresponding to the scheme I have described. We have two
different but parallel teams of workers: the first for social
and rehabilitation problems, the second for methodological and
psychological research.
It seems evident that the experience gained by the first team
can influence the research and clinical activity of the second,
while the experimentation and evalutations of the second guide
the work of the first, creating a "two way" feed back which
can guarantee a theoretical and pratical permanence of the
activity.
On this basis we can operate in the following areas:
1) Early age psychopedagogy;
2) Access to reading and writing;
3) Access to autonomous mobility;
4) Psychopodagogical counseling to the family;
5) Educational counseling;
6) Vocational counseling.
As far as reading and writing are concerned, low vision problems can be restricted to those people who can approach by
themselves a very small amount of printed characters, even if
their access to these skills is very much compromised by the
level of residual vision and/or field.
This double and contradictory message is, according to our
experience, what defines a low vision problem, from a psycho-

logical and functional point of view.

Then we have two different and contradictory areas of rehabilitation:

1) Psychological area
   (missed identification as sighted or blind)
   In this area we can observe the fear of who cannot see and the motivation of who could see.
2) Functional area
   We have here a negative diagnosis of minimal residual vision and/or visual field, but a positive trend to utilize these two residual efficiency.

From these two moments a methodological and technological approach takes places:

Usually who comes to our center has already used all the existing traditional optical and ophtalmological resources (lenses, loupes, microscopes and telescopes) and nevertheless cannot read with proficiency: in these cases we consider the opportunity to use a CCTV aid, which we developed as a prototype in two versions (now built and commercialized by an italian firm): a fix version comprehending the camera, a monitor and the x - y table, the second portable (most useful for students) comprehending only the camera and the x - y table, being suitable to be connected with a normal TV.

Methodological set varies however according to ophthalmological diagnosis, functional and social aims and individual needs: we do not think useful here explain the methodological approaches. Anyway it is important to underline that our evalutation parameters have been still now confirmed by our double intervention in psychological and technological aspects.

Infact, as a consequence of our training we observed:

a) from a functional point of view an increasing of:
   1) contextual integration
   2) speech fluency
   3) text comprehension
   4) short term memory;
b) from a psychological point of view an increasing of
   1) motivation
   2) perseverance
   3) capacity of attention;
   and a decreasing of fatigue together with a better muscolar tone.

First results of our research (that is still going on) seem to suggest furthermore that teaching an early use of CCTV and allowing children to familiarize with it, can be of help in filling the gap existing in the development of an efficient eye-hand interaction, and in creating the necessary parallels between objects'concept and its symbolic graphic rapresentation.

As I pointed out, trying to identify new programs which can lead to better global approaches to the problems of low vision

we thought it very important to involve again all the competen
ces required, using a model of team work that we consider essential for the purpose.
We hope it will be possible here to share different experiences
and to favour specific cooperation among the centers of rehabilitation existing in Europe.

REFERENCES

1. Chapman E.K. "Visually handicapped children and young
   people" Routledge and Kegan Paula, London 1978
2. N.C. "The visually handicapped child in school" Lowenfeld
Constable (U.S.A.) 1974

218

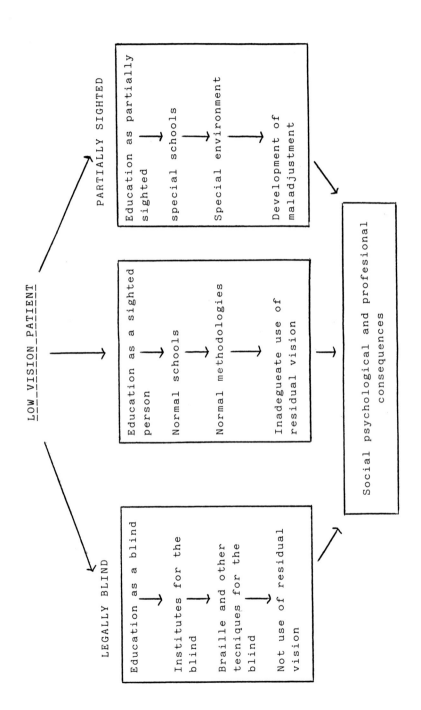

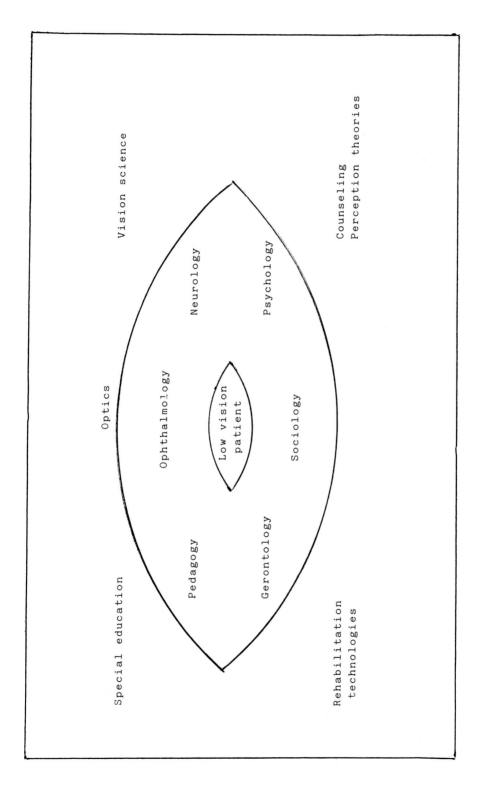

Vision science

Optics

Neurology

Ophthalmology

Psychology

Low vision
patient

Sociology

Pedagogy

Gerontology

Special education

Counseling
Perception theories

Rehabilitation
technologies

METHODOLOGICAL APPROACH

Psychological area (missed identification as sighted or blind) Fear (I cannot see) Motivation (I could see)	Functional area - Diagnosis of minimal residual vision and/or visual field - Positive trend to use the residual efficiency

Increasing in:

1) Motivation
2) Perseverance
3) Capacity of attention

Increasing in:

1) Contextual integration
2) Speech fluency
3) Text comprehension
4) Short-term memory

Decreasing of fatigue

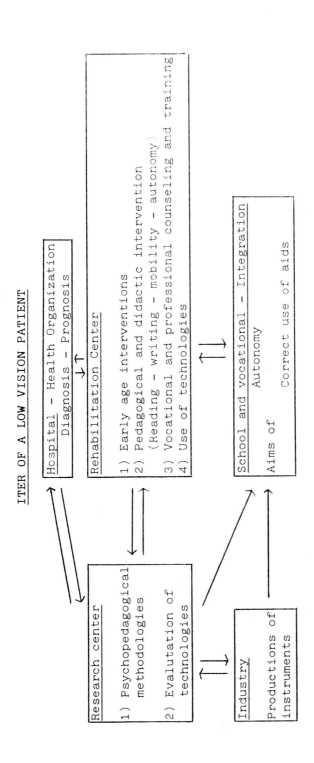

ITER OF A LOW VISION PATIENT

Hospital – Health Organization
Diagnosis – Prognosis

Rehabilitation Center

1) Early age interventions
2) Pedagogical and didactic intervention
   (Reading – writing – mobility – autonomy)
3) Vocational and professional counseling and training
4) Use of technologies

School and vocational – Integration
Autonomy

Aims of
        Correct use of aids

Research center

1) Psychopedagogical
   methodologies

2) Evalutation of
   technologies

Industry

Productions of
instruments

222

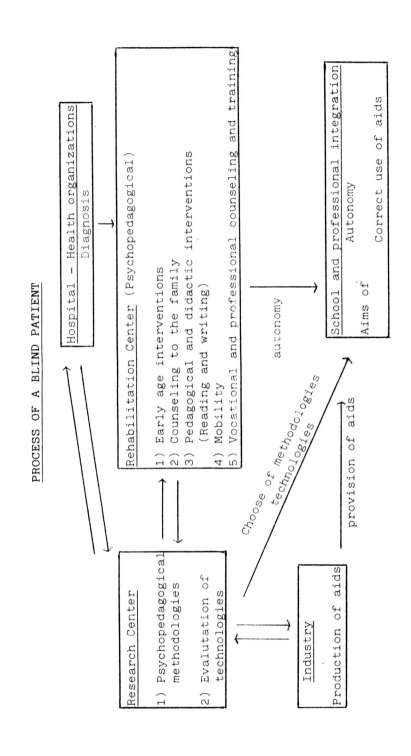

PROCESS OF A BLIND PATIENT

Hospital – Health organizations
Diagnosis

Rehabilitation Center (Psychopedagogical)

1) Early age interventions
2) Counseling to the family
3) Pedagogical and didactic interventions
   (Reading and writing)
4) Mobility
5) Vocational and professional counseling and training

Research Center

1) Psychopedagogical
   methodologies

2) Evalutation of
   technologies

Industry
Production of aids

Choose of methodologies
technologies

autonomy

provision of aids

School and professional integration
Autonomy
Aims of
      Correct use of aids

DISCUSSION

Orban

Perhaps I should introduce myself, since I have not yet delivered my paper. I may be a little bit different from many of you, in
that my research interests are somewhat different. I am a brain
scientist, and I am interested in the cortical mechanisms of visual perception. Now, many of you have probably been impressed
by the quality of the papers in the previous sessions. But many
of you may also have been overwhelmed by the technicality, what
I would call the technicality, of the presentations. I understand, of course, the enthusiam of the engineers about the new
possibilities they have - all these microelectronics, the microprocessors, etc., which have become available. So, many new ho-
rizons open to us. But it may have shifted a little bit the emphasis and the kind of questions we are addressing. I should
really exclude the last two presentations from this remark, but
still I think it is important to make it. I got the impression
yesterday morning, yesterday afternoon and this morning, that in
many instances what people were concerned with, was "what can
machines do". The real question is "what can blind do with them".
I think we needed a little "recentering" in the discussion at
this point. Just recently we had some of this "recentering", but
I thought it was important to make this point. So, the real
problem is to make a useful machine. I will give you just briefly
what is my solution to this problem. It also allows me to introduce something that in my opinion should have been said before.
The main protagonist in this whole game is the brain, and so the
problem becomes "how can we get in the absence of a functioning
visual channel, visual information to the brain?". The problem
has already been tackled a little bit, people have already made
remarks on how many people do use the devices. Some of the devices were extremely complex and difficult to use. In the last
discussion also we had elements of evaluation. So, all this
points to the same problem. It was what Dr. Emiliani called the
"practicability" and I would translate this: How is the aid accepted by the brain? That's the problem. So, I think it's important that we try to devise our aids in such a way that they fit
the rules of the brain. We may have a problem on hand that is
similar to other bioengineering problems where you have artificial implants that are often rejected by the organism. I would
say that the difficulty we have with some aids is just similar.
The last point I want to make is that I am happy that in this
session we have not just engineering contributions, but we also
have contributions from an ophtalmologist and from a psychologist. So, I think, in this "low-vision" session, we may be able
to approach a little more globally the whole problem of visual
handicaps. There will be talks on the different needs of low-

vision patients. That should help us, to some extent, to design
aids. Then, there will be, I guess, a number of aids that will
be reviewed, and finally there will be contributions on the
evaluations of these aids. This last point can then be fed-back,
and help us to improve the design. So, we have not only a multidisciplinary approach, but also one in which we can gradually
improve our aids.

Warburg (to Levett)

I fear that the statistics that you showed us, show very little
about the distribution of the disorders present, but very much
about the conditions of the practitioners of ophtalmology. It
seems that opportunities for electroretinography were very scarce,
since there were so few patients with retinal degenerations on
your tables. It was also apparent that there was little information about multihandicapped children, because there were so few
optic atrophies.

Levett

I do not think I have to say anything more. We are starting from
scratch. The available data is incomplete and that which exists
needs to be examined rigorously. One can probably generalize this
and it constitutes a great difficulty for the development of our
National Health Care System. It strikes me that it is not so much
a problem of ophtalmology but of overall organization and administration of services. In this case, the collection of pertinent
data and the organization of rehabilitation services.

Truquet (to Levett)

You spoke of the transfer of technology, and we have the same problem, when you consider, for example, the work made by Prof. Bruel
and Mr. Lirou. If the transfer is not made, it is because the tactile Braille characters are very expensive and we cannot find a
manufacturer able to produce the device at low cost. We have many
problems as this one.

Levett

I think the technology transfer is a very, very difficult one. One
cannot just transfer technology. One must also transfer the attitudes, etc., to make it work in the local context. This is just
another of our problems. A compatible infrastructure for technology absorption in an optimal or adequate fashion might not be
available. If available, in Greece it is certainly inadequate.
Let me just, as an additional point, say something, that is, in
essence, the technology transfer problem: the Japanese have done
a lot of work on ferrite technology, and they have found a way of
extracting ferrite particles from pollutants, which is of course
a step in the right direction. They have also found a way of

placing these magnetic particles in paints. You all have been
in hospitals in which, running along the walls or on the floor,
is found red, yellow, etc., lines. Someone who is rather confused
will be told to follow the red line which will take him from A
to B, which might be 3 hundred yards, 300 meters. The Japanese
technology can lay down in paint the ferrite particles, and then
use a magnetic probe to follow the line. This could be done without changing the environment. I think, this is one of the problems. We have to provide information, as close as possible, to the
physiological situation. Likewise, we have to provide information
without changing the environment. It's a physical problem. We
know that if we measure in a physical system, the act of measure-
ment itself, gives another system. Therefore, since we do have
lines, here is perhaps an opportunity. The Japanese are in the
process of trying this out, that is laying down the lines of
paint and then developing a magnetic probe for the blind. This
would enable blind persons to find their way in the labyrinth of
a hospital or complicated building going from point A to point B.
It could also be used in streets. I'm sure that one can think of
all kinds of other applications, but this is one interesting aspect of technology transfer.

Question (to Silver)

Do you use strong addition for low-vision people on microscope
systems?

Silver

Yes, certainly dependent on their needs, of course. We routinely
use up to 10 dioptres binocularly with supporting prism if need
be to aid convergence. Higher powers than that I do not find work
binocularly, and I need to go to monocular aids and then we routinely prescribe up to about 12x, but you do run into problems
with lighting at the higher levels.

Orban (to Silver)

You will probably realize that when you have this partial deficit
in your retina, what happens is that your central nervous system
is partially "disafferented". Now we know there are sensory modalities, notably in the tactile system, for which there is experimental evidence that the cortical region that becomes free of
afferents is taken over by other afferents, and we have been in-
vestigating this in the visual system. Now, do you think that,
for example, in a patient who has lost his central vision, he is
able to do more than what a normal patient, or a normal person,
could do with his peripheral retina?

Silver

I really need help from Dr. Warburg. I am not aware that there

is any evidence that the region that is represented by other
modalities takes up spare brain space or even that the peripheral visual receptors in some way move across. It is my understanding that each rod and cone is represented at the visual cortex
individually. What I think is very true is that people learn to
use the degraded information that they get from the peripheral
retina better. Some authorities would claim that people's vision
improves if they use low-vision aids. I'm not sure that their vision improves, but what certainly does improve is their ability
to use that vision.

Warburg

Yes, people learn to scan the texts. They learn to recognize partial information. This is not only the case when you use special
optic aids. If you ask small children who are congenitally visually impaired, they'll tell about the curious clues that they use.
Thus, the v.i. patients use vision in a different way, and very
cleverly.

Orban

Thank you. So, then, if I summarize these two ideas it means that
adaptation is at a very high level.

Question (to Tobin)

It's really two questions. One very simple: can you assume that
your children have stable vision? The second question: can you
tell us what the optimum window size might be for reading?

Tobin

No, to the second one. Yes, to the first. We regularly update
our data bases in terms of the measured visual acuities of the
children. Therefore, when the study is completed, it will be possible for us to look at the relationship between perhaps varying
visual acuities. In other words, all I've done at the moment is
to present means and standard deviations of the group, as a
whole. It will be possible for me to examine the data with a
view to finding out whether there are some who are above the
sighted norms and if so whether they fall within a specified
group. Yes, I think the data will allow me to make that kind of
fine-detailed analysis in due course. I said "no" to the second
one. All I mean is, that I can't specify what the window may be.
I don't know whether the perceptual psychologists can. I think
one way of doing it, as we saw with Dr. King's paper this morning on Braille, is by increasing the number of Braille cells
available, and determine empirically at what point does reading
speed seem to improve.

Soede (to Tobin)

You say, you engineers should think about that, you engineers, etc. Well, I don't think it's the right attitude. You should say: we have to do this, I, myself with the engineer. You have also to take the responsibility for designing aids.

Tobin

Yes, I mean, I couldn't agree with that more fervently. On the other hand, in gatherings like this, it is permissible to go overboard for the sake of provoking people and getting their attention. In a sense, what I'm saying is that engineering groups, whether they are in academic institutions or commercial institutions, ought to recognize that they do need a multidisciplinary approach. And after all I think that in one sense the primary responsibility is there, because they are the people with the ideas about aids. I'm saying that their directors, their fund-givers, ought to build into the team the perceptual psychologists and the educators from the beginning and not leave it to be done later on. But I recognize your point. I'm responsible, and glad to be able to say it, but that doesn't seem to me to be sufficient reason not to use such words as "you engineers".

Silver

If I can come back on this, there is nothing about engineering which enables them to work alone. When I acquired closed-circuit television, the entire hospital was extremely worried about extra insurance, because all I knew about electronics is that if you press the wrong two wires together, everything goes "bang". I think it is the job of the clinicians to identify the problems and of the engineers and the technologists to solve them. And then perhaps for us to run the trials, to evaluate the solutions, and then they go back. We need the interaction, we are totally symbiotic, we need each other.

Tobin

I must spend the rest of the workshop backtracking because I couldn't disagree more strongly with Janet. I want to argue that the educators and psychologists should be part of the team at the design stage. One can design aids even if one is not an engineer, but I think one can do that when he is part of a team. At the moment, we do tend to work in separate boxes: the brain specialist is one, the psychologists in different boxes, the educators in others, the engineers in different kinds of engineering boxes. That's why perhaps a workshop like this is valuable in the sense that it will say what can the E.E.C. do. Perhaps it can insure that there is a drive, a push, towards more collaboration among the disciplines. Perhaps, it can provide the means that the individual countries, the individual academic institutions and firms, seem unable to provide at the moment.

Truquet

The engineers work with the blind and with medical teams in Toulouse. When we produce a device, the blind are there to test the device, and when they say: "We don't like that", we have to bring that modification. It is very important to work with the blind, not only engineers and medical pople, there should be also the blind.

Orban

That's an "a posteriori" mechanism. I think we need to introduce "a priori", into the design of aids.

Warburg

It is curious to see in medicine how the cooperation with technologists arises when the problem is ripe. I need only to refer to what is going on in radiology. No radiological department would be happy without their engineer any more. It's one of the most fashionable examples. Audiology is another one. You will always find a sound engineer there. I think also of the modern chromosomal investigations where you use picture identification and put them on a computer. Now, when the problem is there, cooperation will appear, provided that a structure of the medical speciality is right for the two parties. This is why we have to make visual aids an acceptable part of ophtalmology, something that will give merit to the people involved.It's also important to create a name for this cooperative study - audiology is fine for hearing. I would like pople to accept this part of medicine as something of special importance and in that case cooperation will appear immediately, I'm sure.

Levett

I think that what we have to avoid is when the psychologist will tell us and insist that it was the cat that sat on the floor, the engineer comes back and says: "No, the cat sat in the flower" - which is a possibility. The thing is that it is hard to define how problems are solved and it's much more difficult to define our complex problems ourselves. There is no exact methodology of going about it. It's a matter of people who are interested in a particular problem coming together with the right kinds of knowledge relative to that problem, and coming up with a solution or alternative solutions. I think that bioengineering - some people would argue that it is not a discipline -, but nevertheless I think it is demonstrative of that bridge between the physical sciences and the medical sciences that leads to certain kinds of solutions. It's a matter of communication, in terms of passing information back and forth, so that the solutions can be worked out.

Tobin

May I just give a specific example of this kind of problem?
It's a very small one, but it's a serious one. There wasn't a
proper collaboration between, on the one hand, the engineer with
the device and the teacher working with blind children. In
Britain, there is an engineer who has come up with a device that
will allow grade 1 Braille to be output on tape very quickly
and easily. He was very pleased with this and I went along to
have a look at it, and said: "Well, that's very interesting, but
how is the teacher who is watching what the child is reading
going to be able to read this Braille by sight, because you have
got it only in one colour, and if you try to read Braille by
sight, you will know the importance of getting the page at the
right angle so that the shadow is properly cast, so that you can
see the dots". Now, a teacher cannot be of great assistance to a
learner until he knows what it is that is under the child's fingers, or what has just gone under. It's a simple case, and it
can be solved using a different material that would cast a shadow or that would provide a contrast between the figure, the
Braille dots, and the ground upon which it existed. Now, it's
easily solved if there is the simplest kind of collaboration.

Emiliani

I think this is one of the main points of this workshop. The
importance of the workshop is to try and find, if possible, some
ways so that in multinational and multidisciplinary organizations
it is possible to start a new way of thinking about aids, starting from the needs of the people and discussing about these needs,
proposing different approaches to solve the problems and then,
hopefully, finding the solutions which can be technical or not.
We have to find, not what can separate the different persons,
but some common ground and then from this common ground to construct this new communication for the development of aids.

Question (to Tobin)

If I understood you correctly, one of the conclusions of your
contribution is that, on one hand, by magnifying the image, you
win in acuity, but you lose in a number of other points, that
is in reduction in the number of possible scanning strategies,
and in field size, where you have more volatile and short-term
memory. Then, would it be possible to make an evaluation to test
these different factors and to see whether you come up to some
optimum where you have the maximum gain in acuity and the minimum losses?

Tobin

Yes, there must be. I have not investigated the trade-off, because we are at the very preliminary stages of development here.

It's essentially a problem in the earlier stages of learning,
the one you are able to cope with. This isn't a problem for you,
and I think the developmental aspect of it needs to be looked at.
I've been also asking myself whether there are similar problems
vis-à-vis the 65 and 70 years old and 75 years old. Perhaps
there is a gradual deterioration in short-term memory capacity
that we should bear in mind when we are designing aids, perhaps
by, for example, multiplying the number of channels which they
can use, and perhaps just by being aware of the fact that if you
increase the magnification to this extent, you're now beginning
to invoke some other kinds of problems. I don't know if I've
answered your question. Your point is in the right direction,
but I think that we ought to bear in mind with the visually
handicapped child that things like short-term memory do go on
developing to the age of about 12. I mean, my own research has
shown that at age 5, for example, the totally blind perform
better on digit and letter span tests than those with better
sight. Now, I think that's interesting and can be parsimoniously
interpreted in terms of the fact they practise and reach their
potential, full potential, earlier, and so we could capitalize
on that. When we are talking about the low-vision child, we are
talking about a child perhaps who hasn't improved his short-term
memory capacity through practice, and we are making things more
difficult for him. However, the child has such a power of accommodation in his eyes and can vary the distance of the object,
which allows him also to increase and decrease the size of the
field. I'm a great optimist at heart.

Silver

I would like to add here two small observations that I can't
support with a great deal of objective research. We've got a
large group of people now who are using close circuit TV as an
aid to employment, and I've recorded the optimum magnification
levels when the aids were prescribed in the clinic. I'm now
talking about groups that run into some hundreds of subjects.
We've always prescribed a minimum magnification level, the
minimum magnification level that was possible, in order to give
as large an area on the screen as possible. But when these patients returned to the clinic, and we asked them to adjust the
instrument to the magnification level that they are then using,
they are almost without exception choosing higher levels of
magnification than were selected at the original assessment.
The same sort of things tend to happen with children in reverse.
When you first prescribe for a child, they seem to require
rather high levels of magnification, in other words, you seem
to need to make the task visually easy. Then, at a later stage,
when they've learned the skill of using the aids, I am often
able to reduce the magnification level. Now, I don't know enough

about perception and psychology to interpret these results. I'm
putting them into the pot as clinical observations for other
people to make what they will of them.

Thomsen

So far we've been talking about the perceptual approach to reading. Now, there are other approaches to reading and by that I
mean that when I set up my strategies for reading a text, I ask
myself what is the aim of reading that text, what information am
I looking for in the text. Now, there are many strategies you can
set up when you have the book in front of you. We've had experiences in Denmark with students, some with good vision and some
with very low vision. Those with rather good vision had an ex-
traordinary low reading speed, less than 100 words per minute,
and there were no perceptual reasons why they should have such a
low reading speed. So we tried to set up programs to teach them
these other strategies, together with students with very low vision, 2 or 3 over 60, who had a very low reading speed as well
because of perceptual reasons. Now both groups read at a reading
speed greater than the normally sighted students, say 300 to 400
words per minute. Because they didn't know how to read, not from
a perceptive point of view, but from a more psychological point
of view. I think we should be aware of these other approaches to
reading when we talk about both low-vision readers or partially
sighted readers, and Braille readers as well.

Session 4: TRANSDUCTION OF VISUAL INFORMATION AND DISPLAYS FOR THE BLIND

Chairman: D.J. Powell

Transitory Graphical Displays for the Blind
J.M. Gill

The Computer as a Graphical Communication Tool for the Blind
P. Graziani

Image Processing Techniques: Some Possible Applications to the Transduction of Visual Information to Other Modalities
D.J. Powell

Design of Sensory Substitution Systems for the Blind
C. Veraart, G.A. Orban, M.C. Wanet, I. Richard

Discussion

TRANSITORY GRAPHICAL DISPLAYS FOR THE BLIND

J.M. Gill
Research Unit for the Blind, Brunel University
Uxbridge, Middlesex, England

There is a need for hardcopy and transitory graphical displays for the blind. However relatively little is known about the optimum presentation of graphical information in a non-visual form, particularly for multi-modal displays.

Most computer-related aids for the blind are for conveying textual or numerical information by tactile or auditory displays. These displays may be time invariant such as braille embossed on paper, or be transitory such as a refreshable braille display of raised pins. However there is much information which sighted people have presented in graphical form which is difficult to present clearly in textual form to the visually handicapped.

The conventional approach is to use an embossed map or diagram, with the text displayed as braille. Variation in the type and elevation of point, line and areal symbols can facilitate the tactual reading of a graphical display. For instance Schiff, Kaufer and Mosak (1966) showed that a line saw-tooth in cross-section can be useful for conveying directional information since the line is smooth in one direction and rough in the other.

Of the thirty systems that have been developed for producing embossed maps and diagrams for the blind (Gill, 1974), most are very labour intensive and therefore expensive if paid staff are employed. The problem is exasperated by the optimum conversion from a visual presentation to a tactual one being more of an art than a science. At present this conversion requires human intervention in all but the simplest graphical representations.

Here is an obvious application for computer-aided design; the task has similarities to the preparation of artwork for integrated circuit masks or a multi-layered printed circuit board. One such system was developed some years ago (Gill, 1973), and it has been further developed by Clark and Balsam (1982) and Fries (1983).

This system uses conventional interactive graphics on a visual display unit for the design stage, and the computer then controls an engraving machine to produce a negative master. A positive is made in epoxy, and plastic copies are vacuum formed from the positive master.

This system produces good quality tactual output but it would be improved if the computer could directly generate the embossed map or diagram. However this would only "solve" part of the problem. There is an increasing requirement for a refreshable non-visual graphics display.

There are about six paperless braille devices commercially available (Gill, 1984), but they all have a single line of braille display. Maure (Foulke, 1981) and Rose (1979) are developing page braille displays which will have advantages over line displays for tabular material and simple graphics. However there is a limit to the amount of graphical information that can be displayed with evenly-spaced single-elevation dots.

This problem will become more acute with increasing use by the blind of digital information systems. For instance the British Telecom Prestel viewdata system can now be output in braille (Gill, 1981); this is just the alphanumeric data with the graphics being ignored. This type of system will be much easier to use when page braille displays are commercially available at a reasonable price.

The problem is not only one of hardware but also software since the optimum conversion is likely to require a complex algorithm.

If the text is displayed in braille it does not mean that the graphics must be in a tactual form. For instance one could consider a display which uses both auditory and tactual stimuli. Such a proposal is not new but little research has been done in this area. One possible configuration would a x-y plate which when touched gives an audible signal which varies in frequency and amplitude according to two dependent variables at that x-y coordinate.

Before designing such a display it is important to ascertain the factors which determine ease of use by a blind person. This is a far from trivial task which has received comparatively little attention.

Research has been mainly concentrated on audio displays partly because they are much easier to design and build. Pollack and Ficks (1954) studied multi-dimensional auditory displays in which each variable had only two states. They found that, in general, multiple stimulus encoding is a satisfactory procedure for increasing the information transmission rate associated with such displays.

Roffler and Butler (1968a) found that listeners could locate auditory stimuli accurately in the vertical plane when the stimulus was complex and included frequencies above 7kHz. Roffler and Butler (1968b) then found that subjects tended to place the audio stimuli on a vertical scale in accordance with their respective pitch. Higher-pitched sounds were perceived as originating above lower-pitched sounds.

A variety of two dimensional auditory displays have been built; for instance Black (1968) developed a display where the horizontal coordinate was represented by time delay and amplitude of the signal and the vertical coordinate by frequency (100-400 Hz). Fish and Beschle (1973) also used frequency (200-7000 Hz) for representing the vertical position of the scan but interaural differences (up to 40 dB) for the horizontal.

Phillips and Seligman (1974) developed a multi-dimensional auditory display in which frequency, amplitude and timbre are all utilised. Robinson (Gill, 1975) also developed a two dimensional display, where the frequency of the signal depends on the vertical coordinate and time delay for the horizontal. However there has been little systematic comparison of the various types of auditory displays even though Kramer (1962) mentioned the need for this nearly two decades ago.

Davall and Gill (1975 & 1977) developed two performance parameters for assessing displays but they would be difficult to apply in practice to multi-modal displays.

That the foregoing has been more a catalogue of problems rather than solutions reflects the lack of research on computer-generated graphics displays for the blind. It is important that the next generation of displays are scientifically designed to be optimum for the user and not just the easiest to manufacture.

References

Black W L "An Acoustic Pattern Presentation". Research Bulletin of the American Foundation for the Blind, No 16, May 1968, pp 93-132.

Clark L L & Balsam M "The Baruch College Tactual Graphics Facility: A Progress Report". Braille Research Newsletter, No 13, June 1982, pp 34-37.

Davall P W & Gill J M "A Method for the Comparative Evaluation of Visual and Auditory Displays". Research Bulletin of the American Foundation for the Blind, No 29, June 1975, pp 9-21.

Davall P W & Gill J M "A Comparison of Human Operator Transient Response to Visual and Auditory Displays". American Foundation for the Blind Research Report, ISBN 0 89128 952 6, 1977, 27 pp.

Fish R M & Beschle R G "An Auditory Display Capable of Presenting Two Dimensional Shapes to the Blind". Research Bulletin of the American Foundation for the Blind, No 26, June 1973, pp 5-18.

Foulke E "Braille Research in the Perceptual Alternatives Laboratory". Braille Research Newsletter, No 12, 1981,

238

Fries P "A New CAM System for Tactual Graphics". Braille Research Newsletter, No 14, July 1983, pp 14-17.

Gill J M "Design, Production and Evaluation of Tactual Maps for the Blind". PhD Thesis, University of Warwick, 1973.

Gill J M "Tactual Mapping". Research Bulletin of the American Foundation for the Blind, No 28, Oct 1974, pp 57-80.

Gill J M "Auditory and Tactual Displays for Sensory Aids for the Visually Impaired". Research Bulletin of the American Foundation for the Blind, No 29, June 1975, pp 187-196.

Gill J M "Microprocessor Braille Systems". Computers and Braille Conference, Toulouse, France, Sept 1981.

Gill J M "International Survey of Aids for the Visually Disabled". Research Unit for the Blind, Brunel University, 1984, ISBN 0 902215 57 4, 121 pp.

Kramer H J "Stimulus Variables in Auditory Projective Testing". Research Bulletin of the American Foundation for the Blind, No 1, Jan 1962, pp 33-40.

Phillips J A & Seligman P M "Two Instruments for the Blind Engineer". Research Bulletin of the American Foundation for the Blind, No 27, April 1974, pp 187-216.

Pollack I & Ficks L "Information of Elementary Multi-dimensional Auditory Displays". Journal of the Acoustical Society of America, Vol 26, No 2, March 1954, pp 155-158.

Roffler S K & Butler R A "Factors that Influence the Localisation of Sound in the Vertical Plane". Journal of the Acoustical Society of America, Vol 43, No 6, 1968, pp 1255-9.

Roffler S K & Butler R A "Localisation of Tonal Stimuli in the Vertical Plane". Journal of the Acoustical Society of America, Vol 43, No 6, 1968, pp 1260-6.

Rose L "Full-Page Paperless Braille Display". Braille Research Newsletter, No 10, 1979, pp 59-60.

Schiff W, Kaufer L & Mosak S "Informative Tactile Stimuli in the Perception of Direction". Perceptual and Motor Skills, No 23, Monogr Suppl 7, 1966.

Author's note: This paper is based on one presented by the author at the conference on Uses of Computers in Aiding the Disabled held in Haifa in 1981.

THE COMPUTER AS A GRAPHICAL COMMUNICATION TOOL FOR THE BLIND

P. Graziani
Istituto di Ricerca sulle Onde Elettromagnetiche (I.R.O.E.)
Consiglio Nazionale delle Ricerche (C.N.R.)
Via Panciatichi 64, 50127 Firenze, Italy

The aim of this report is to propose the computer as a tool for the blind to communicate, process and receive graphical information.

A blind person usually receives and communicate verbally even if, in many cases, a drawing would be a more effective form of communication. This is due to the difficulty to make available for the blind tactile images of good quality and to produce drawings, by the blind themselves, to communicate information to other people.

Three different ways of using a computer to increase the possibilities of graphical communication for the blind are suggested here.

1) Interactive reading of a tactile image

A typical example of a tactile image is represented by a mobility map. It is well known that a tactile map cannot provide as much information as a visual map [1]. In addition, there are many problems of discriminability of the various kinds of information. Braille scripts and special tactile symbols, which are necessary to add information in the map, are often an obstacle to the perception of the shapes and the general structure of the map.

The amount and discriminability of information can be enlarged by using a computer-aided reading procedure by means of a digitizing graphics tablet, a suitable software and a multimodal display. In this case, the tactile information present in the map can be reduced to only the contours of the shapes, such as buildings, route configurations, etc. Such a "clean" map allows good discrimination of the shapes while, all the other information, related to each point of the map, can be provided, directly by the computer, in another form such as synthetic speech or paperless Braille. This latter kind of information is not limited by the little space available in the map; it can be very detailed and may be recalled by entering the coordinates of the point by means of the stylus of the digitizing tablet.

The computer could also suggest in which direction the stylus has to be moved to reach a requested point, for example: a square, a street, a building, a bus stop, etc.

Such a "talking map" would consist in a tactile map and in a corresponding data file in the computer.

The reading procedure could be as follows: put the tactile map onto the digitizing graphics tablet; load the interactive reading program with the corresponding data file; reset the framework of the interactive reading program to establish the 1 to 1 relation between the tactile map and the corresponding software image in the computer (for example, by entering the coordinates of the four corners of the map); then it is possible to recall any information related to a point of the map by means of the stylus of the graphics tablet.

Such a kind of map can be designed with a computer-aided technique similar to those developed to design tactile maps [2],[3].

A tactile version of the map can be obtained by means of one of the optical-to-tactile conversion systems [4],[5] available today, from a drawing produced by the computer. The tactile version can also be produced directly by the computer if a tactile graphical peripheral is available. Moreover, it is possible to organize the information related to other kinds of tactile images, such as geographical maps and graphics used in science. For example, it is possible to obtain, with great accuracy, the coordinates of any point of a XY line graph, without the need of an additional tactile grid [6].

A computer equipped with a multimodal display (digitizing tablet, speech synthesizer and interactive tactile reading software), as described here, could be a powerful general communication aid for the blind. For instance, it could be applied to programmed instruction and even to develop some kinds of computer games for the blind.

2) Optical-to-tactile conversion

Another application of the computer to problems related to tactile images is to enlarge and improve the possibilities of optical to tactile conversion.

Image processing techniques [7], such as edge detection, line thinning, etc., can be used to obtain a clear tactile version of black and white drawings.

Incidentally, we may note that this kind of image processing, if implemented on-line into the Optacon process, would improve the reading performance in case of poor quality of print or types of characters difficult to read, such as heavy type.

Other image processing techniques, such as image segmentation and following of contours, can be used to obtain a satisfactory tactile version even of some kinds of simple pictures [8]. For example, it is possible to transform a picture into a simplified image, with few gray levels; each region with a homogenous gray level can be represented with its contour or with a synthetic texture.

These techniques cannot generally solve the problem of a tactile version of pictures but, in many cases, they allow a blind person to perceive at least some features of the image that can be useful to understand a text when the picture is inserted in it as a significant part.

3) Computer graphics for the blind

Blind people are able to construct mental images which are much more complex than those they can actually produce on paper because the tools available for the blind allow to draw only simple images.

A special computer-aided graphics technique can improve very much the possibility to draw for the blind.

By using a suitable software and a computer equipped with a speech synthesizer, graphics screen and graphics printer, the blind user can develop a drawing composed, for example, of a number of simple elements, such as triangles, squares, circles, single segments, Braille or normal characters and other symbols.

The mental image of the drawing can be decomposed in a sequence of such simple elements and data related to each of them, i.e. size and spatial location, can be entered into the computer through the keyboard by the blind themselves.

We may note that this procedure for the construction and analysis of mental images, is a useful exercise that can help a blind child to develop topological and geometrical concepts and the ability to communicate by means of images, especially if the computer makes available a sensory feedback consisting in a tactile version of the drawing by which the child can verify the results of his or her construction.

However, once the procedure has become familiar, it can be extended also to develop drawings which are too complex to be verified, by touch, in their tactile version. In this case, some partial verification can be sufficient to make the blind person able to communicate complex graphical information to a sighted person.

This method for developing two-dimensional drawings, can also be applied to develop a three-dimensional scene. In this case, each single element of the scene can be represented by means of a spatial lattice of segments. For example, we can think of a parallelepiped as consisting of eight points, corresponding to the eight corners, connected by twelve segments.

Data related to each object can include size, orientation and location in space.

Once data are entered into the computer, it is possible to produce drawings, consisting in orthogonal or axonometric projections. It is also possible to produce simulations of a perspective view by choosing the location of the point of view and the direction and opening of the cone of view. In this case, only the parts of the scene which are within the solid angle of such a simulated vision are projected.

242

By means of a tactile version of the images produced by the computer with these procedures, a blind person can also understand how an object, designed by him or her, is transformed by the projection process.

Applications of the computer to problems of graphical communication for the blind are studied in a subproject on Communication Aids of the Special Project on Biomedical and Clinical Engineering of the C.N.R.

Some simple image processing techniques have been applied to obtain a tactile version of pictures.

Some experimental procedures of computer graphics for the blind have been developed [9]. Particular attention has been devoted to the development of a special editor to design two-dimensional and three-dimensional scenes. By using the speech synthesizer as an aid, a blind person can create each object of the scene by entering data corresponding to the points and connections between these points. A scene is composed with a number of these simple objects. Each object is labelled and can be recalled through this label in order to be corrected, inserted, deleted, translated or rotated into the scene. The union of two or more objects to create a new complex object is also possible.

Drawings are produced on the screen of the computer and in hard copy by means of a graphics printer.

Also, an embossing paper plotter is being developed to obtain computer-controlled tactile drawings.

These studies are carried out in cooperation with the research group on Special Education of the Institute for the Blind in Milan and the Printing House for the Blind of the Regional Administration of Tuscany.

References

[1]   G. Jansson: "Tactual maps as a challenge for perception research"; Paper read at the First International Symposium in Maps and Graphics for Visually Handicapped: Ass. of American Geographers, Washington, D.C., March 1983.

[2]   J.M. Gill, L.L. Clark: "Resources for creating tactual graphics"; J. of Visual Impairment and Blindness, vol. 72, no. 1, pp. 32-33, January 1978.

[3]   L.L. Clark, M. Balsam: "The Baruch College tactual graphics facility: a progress report"; Braille Research Newsletter, no. 13, pp. 34-37, June 1982.

[4]   R. Erhardt, H. Offner, M. Schlipf, P. Schwarzmann: "Fast and economic conversion of images to a tactile presentation for blind people"; Medical Progress through Technology, vol. 6, pp. 123-130, 1979.

[5]   "Stereo copier"; Braille Research Newsletter, no. 13, pp. 21, June 1982.

[6]   S.J. Lederman, J.I. Campbell: "Tangible line graphs: an
       evaluation of some systematic strategies for exploration";
       J. of Visual Impairment and Blindness, vol. 77, no. 3, pp.
       108-112, March 1983.
[7]   W.K. Pratt: "Digital image processing"; J. Wiley ed., New
       York, 1978.
[8]   T. Pun: "Tactile artificial sight: segmentation of images
       for scene simplification"; IEEE Biomedical Engineering,
       vol. BME 29, no. 4, pp. 293-299, April 1982.
[9]   P. Graziani, C. Susini: "Grafica con il calcolatore orien-
       tata ai non vedenti"; Paper presented at the Conf. on
       "Ausili per handicap di comunicazione" (Communication aids),
       IROE - CNR, March 1983.

IMAGE PROCESSING TECHNIQUES: SOME POSSIBLE APPLICATIONS TO THE TRANSDUCTION OF VISUAL INFORMATION TO OTHER MODALITIES

D.J. Powell
Moorfields Eye Hospital
City Road
London EC1V 2PD

Image processing techniques may be classified in terms of a rather loose notion of complexity. Firstly, there are bulk transformations where the one image is translated into another by applying the same rule to each pixel in the source image. Examples of this type of process are differentiation and spatial summation. This type of process is amenable to parallel computation. At a slightly higher level is feature detection: the selection of points satisfying some criteria. Examples of this type of process are the search for and classification of edges, ends of lines, corners and forks. At the next level evaluation may concern compound structures: the spatial relation of simple features to form a new identity. The relations that may be used are to the right of, above, next to, enclosed by etc. For example a square is an edge which is closed, with four corners, and each corner is approximately 90 degrees: a tea cup in profile might be defined by a square next to a circle. Another issue is the handling of the amount of information involved in image processing. An image potentially contains a large amount of information. A picture 512 by 512 pixels with 8 bit colour definition in red, green, and blue will take 0.75 Megabytes of storage. This is roughly equivalent to the storage needed for a book. The human eye scans a picture concentrating on the dominant features and spending variable amounts of time extracting information from the various regions of a scene. Image processing may do likewise by constructing a list of compound structures and storing these as data-base items. Features of a certain type may be rapidly retrieved from such a storage system. Pictures may be compared and recognised by a comparison of such lists of structures rather than by an attempt to match the raw images.

The question of perception of depth is important in many applications. This is a problem in image processing and is all the more troublesome in robotic systems where depth information is required in real time. It seems difficult to achieve the generality of depth perception which is attained by so many living creatures. Particular solutions to the problem involve: the movement of a spot of light over the 3-dimensional scene; varying the viewing position continuously; and searching for corresponding points in two views taken at different angles.

Having discussed some of the techniques of image processing, some consideration can now be given to the type visual impairment. The case of complete loss of visual sensation must, of course, be considered but it should be remembered that loss of visual function may be selective. Loss of central foveal vision will deprive the subject of ability to analyse fine detail within a small angle of view. Loss of peripheral vision entails reduction in sensitivity to movement and to the analysis of gross features. Where loss is selective it makes sense to utilise the visual function that remains and to avoid unnecessarily transducing this surviving information and to concentrate on the extraction of features that the visual system can no longer provide. This implies not only different optical systems for the cameras but also different image processing techniques.

Consider the problem of the transduction of a view of a scene: where for the purposes of this section let a view be defined as that information derived from a single fixation point in a scene. As a rather facile comment let us note that view is not time varying: given sufficient processing power a view can be processed, in human terms, instantaneously. A sound, for example, by its very nature is a variation of displacement with time. A mapping from the visual to the auditory is a mapping of a instantaneous spatial pattern to a time-varying stimulus. A number of choices have to be made when attempting to map visual information into another modality. The correct choice is that which produces the easiest comprehension for an individual. There can be no unique solution: we have already discussed that, apart from total blindness, areas of loss may vary with disease and the solution may be tailored to a particular type of loss. In addition, the rate at which information can be processed may act as a constraint on the complexity of the stimulus presented in any modality. Is the target modality capable of preserving the 2 or 3 dimensional aspects of a view? With good equipment sound can, as can vibration. Both, however, can carry information that has no spatial content. Should the transduction employ direct spatial cues? If so would the normal functioning of the modality be completely disrupted? Can a view be translated into another modality and have a stationary expression. eg. a view corresponds to a chord. This may be too limiting. It may be necessary to scan a view in some elemental way: radial, raster, spiral or annular; and each of these elements to be processed sequentially to provide a cyclical time-varying stimulus. Further more subtle questions concern the complexity of the image and the complexity of the derived parameters. For example, if scanning elements, radial might be preferred to horizontal on grounds of complexity. A similar consideration is the relation between object invariance and parameter invariance. Once more radial might be preferred to horizontal in that edges remain constant despite rotation.

Even these fairly superficial observations seem to indicate that the raster scan imposed by television electronics may less attractive than a radial scan. The radial scan can be easily implemented with image processing facilities.

As a demonstration of this approach consider the following scheme. A radius with centre C moves with constant angular velocity. The radius is divide into 2 equal parts. Those pixels of the scene which lie under the inner half of the radius are averaged to give intensity I1. Similarly the outer half produces and average I2. Suppose we are able to control the loudness of 3 tones. Let V1, V2 and V3 denote the loudness of these tones. The pitch of these tones are constant and increase from tone 1 to tone tone 3.

The following scheme for translating pixel intensity into sound has some attractions.

$d=I2-I1$

$V1=abs(d)$

$V2=$ a if d greater than 0

    0 if d less than or equal to 0

$V3=$ c at one point on the circumference

    0 elsewhere

where a and c are constants. V3 is designed to give orientation.

The sound stimulus can be simplified by temporal smoothing by using:

$V1(t)=d/2+V1(t-1)/2$

This simple system is capable of demonstration.

DESIGN OF SENSORY SUBSTITUTION SYSTEMS FOR THE BLIND

C. Veraart[1x], G.A. Orban[2], M.C. Wanet[1], I. Richard[1]
1 Lab. Neurophysiologie, Université Catholique de Louvain,
  UCL 5449, B-1200 Brussels, Belgium
2 Lab. Neuro- en Psychofysiologie, Katholieke Universiteitte Leuven,
  Campus Gasthuisberg, B-3000 Leuven, Belgium
x Research associate, NFSR, Belgium

Many efforts have been devoted to the design of sensory aids
for blind persons. Since the introduction of Braille last
century, a classical way has been to use the remaining sensory
systems (mainly the auditory and tactile systems) as
substitutive input to the brain. Recent developments in
electronics and computer-science have made possible the design
of sophisticated sensory and artificial substitution systems.
An alternative approach, pioneered by Brindley and Lewin
(1968), has been to bypass the impaired visual receptor organ
(eye) by electrical stimulation of the visual cortex.

The purpose of the present report is to use the organization of
the sensory systems as a guide to develop a unified framework
for these different sensory aids. Comparison of the different
aids within this framework leads us to propose that sensory
substitution systems are potentially the most complete aids and
allows us to derive the conditions for their optimal design.

Development of such optimally designed sensory substitution
systems seems highly desirable given the small proportion of
blind people using aids and the long training periods required
to use the existing aids with success. These two observations
indicate that the major problem in the design of sensory aids
for blind is one of compatibility : how can we make the
substitutive information acceptable for the brain. An
additional motivation for such developments are the limitations
in the rehabilitation achieved by the presently available aids
: they only substitute for text reading and avoidance of
obstacles. Therefore blind people are still deprived of many
aspects of visual perception, such as face recognition so
important in social communication.

THE SENSORY CHANNELS

Although each sensory channel has its own specific features,
due to the different energies to be transduced, one is struck
by the similarities in functioning and organization principles
of the more central parts of these channels as e.g. lateral
inhibition, topographic and columnar organization, multiple
cortical representations. As an example, the visual channel is
organized both serially and in parallel (Fig. 1). At the first
level the light is transduced into nervous energy by the
photoreceptors. These signals are processed by the visual
system including the pathways between the retina and the visual
cortex as well as a number of visual cortical areas surrounding

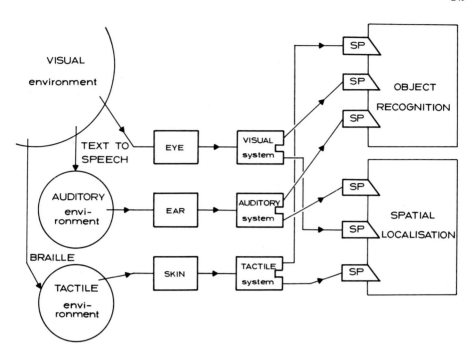

Fig. 1. Three levels of functioning of sensory channels. SP : modality specific parts of the perceptual functions. The manipulation done by the off-line techniques (Braille and text-to-speech) are indicated.

the primary visual cortex (area 17). At different levels in this system parallel processing has been demonstrated (see Orban 1984 for review). Within the retino-geniculo-cortical pathway different functional channels funnel information in parallel to the cortex (ON/OFF center cells, X, Y & W cells, wavelength specific and wavelength non-specific cells). In addition to the direct retino-geniculo-cortical pathway, a second route over the colliculus superior and the pulvinar carries information from the retina to the cortex. At the primary cortical level the different receptive field types analyze the incoming thalamic signals in parallel. Very recently Livingstone and Hubel (1984) have shown a parallel processing of cytochrome-oxydase positive and negative regions between V1 and V2 of the monkey. It has been proposed (Macko et al., 1982) that the visual information flowing through the visual cortical areas splits into two main directions : inferotemporal and parietal cortex, supposedly corresponding to the 2 main perceptual functions of the visual channel : object recognition (what) and spatial localization (where).

Although they have not been investigated in the same detail as the visual channel, the auditory and tactile channels seem to be organized in a similar fashion, whereby transduction and processing lead both to "object" recognition and spatial

250

localization. We suggest that these two perceptual functions
comprise a first modality specific process, corresponding e.g.
in the visual modality to the 3D level of Marr (1982), followed
by an amodal symbolic level (Richard et al., 1983). The three
levels of hierarchy (Fig. 1) in the sensory channels suggest a
similar architecture for the artificial sensory systems
comprising a transducer corresponding to the receptor organ, a
decoder corresponding to the sensory processing system, and
finally an interpreter corresponding to the perceptual
functions.

THE CLASSES OF SENSORY AIDS

The simplest sensory aids as Braille reading and text-to-
speech, only involve an off-line manipulation of the
environment whereby visual information is translated into
auditory or tactile information, which is then processed
normally by the corresponding sensory channel (Fig. 1). In case
of Braille reading, the normal pattern recognition abilities of
the tactile channel are used allowing considerable improvement
with learning. These off-line techniques put the blinds in a
passive receiving situation preventing them to have a direct
access to the environment. Technological developments however
have made possible on-line sensory aids allowing the subject to
interact with the environment.

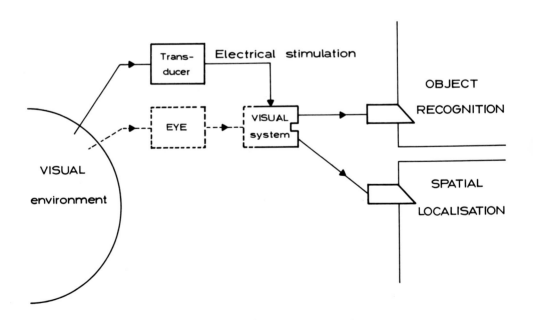

Fig. 2. Direct electrical stimulation of the visual cortex.

One type of on-line techniques bypasses the impaired receptor organ (eye) by direct <u>electrical stimulation of the visual cortex</u> (Brindley and Lewin, 1968; Dobelle et al., 1979). In these visual prostheses the image picked-up by a television camera is digitized and transduced into electrical stimulation of an array of implanted metal electrodes positioned against the visual cortex, resulting in phosphenes perceived by the subject (Fig. 2). In addition to being invasive, this technique has two shortcomings. First, in as much as visual processing starts in the retina, the retinal and geniculate levels of processing are bypassed. Second the subject lacks a reafference signal (von Holst and Mittelstaedt, 1950) resulting in an instability of the phosphenes during eye movements. Theoretically these problems could be solved by processing the visual image before transduction to electrical stimulation. This processing would include modelling the first stages of processing in the retina and the LGN and shifting the images with the eye movements.

A first class of non-invasive on-line techniques, <u>the artificial substitution systems</u>, aim at translating visual information into another sensory information without any reference to the normal functioning of the visual system (Fig. 3). In the Optacon (Nye and Bliss, 1970) the visual information is processed up to recognition of the letter, using algorithms that do not model the visual system and the shape of the letter is then reproduced on the skin by an array of needles without any inverse decoding of the symbol. This

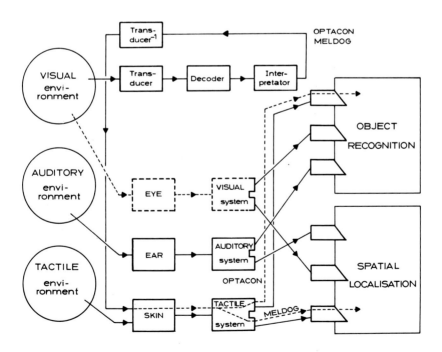

Fig. 3. Artificial substitution systems : Optacon and Meldog.

252

system is only concerned with a limited part of object recognition, namely text reading. The Meldog (Tachi et al., 1982), functions according to similar principles but subserves a spatial localization function. Unless the artificial substitution system would be adaptative, a complete processing leading to recognition of any object or visual scene seems excluded. Even if such a goal were to be achieved it will be at expense of a delay introduced in the transmission to the substitutive channel, loosing the benefit of on-line processing. One wonders how such a system with which the subject has only limited interactions, will be accepted by blind persons.

The second class of non-invasive on-line sensory aids are the sensory substitution systems (Fig. 4). Our definition of sensory substitution is more restricted than that initially proposed by Bach-y-Rita (1972). Contrary to Bach-y-Rita we propose that the neuronal mechanisms involved in sensory substitution are restricted to levels where the convergence between the different sensory channels occur normally, i.e. at the level of the amodal perceptual systems. There is very little evidence for connections between different sensory channels at lower levels, other than those carrying aspecific arrousal type of signals. In addition adult plasticity at the cortical level is limited (Kaas et al., 1983) to compensation of small defects within the channel and it seems unlikely that in an adult organism one channel could massively take over afferents of another one. Since in our hypothesis the neuronal

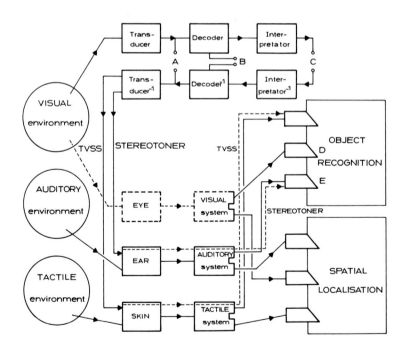

Fig. 4 Sensory substitution systems : tactile vision substitution system (TVSS) and stereotoner.

convergence underlying substitution occurs at the amodal
perceptual level, an optimally designed sensory substitution
system (SSS) should deliver at that level, but through the
substitutive sensory channel e.g. the auditory channel (E in
Fig. 4), the same information as normally delivered by a
non-impaired visual channel (D in Fig. 4). In order to do so
the SSS has first to generate a signal carrying this
information. This is achieved by modelling as closely as
possible the visual channel. After transduction modelling the
eye, the information is processed by a decoder modelling the
visual system and an interpreter modelling the specific stage
of the perceptual functions yielding the required signal (C in
Fig. 4). The second step is to carry this signal to the
amodal perceptual system, through a given substitutive channel
e.g. the auditory channel. This involves modelling the
substitutive channel and inversing the information flow. In
this part of the SSS, signals provided by an inverse
interpreter would be coded by an inverse decoder to be
transduced into an auditory signal, then delivered and
processed by the auditory channel. As a result the visual
prosthesis will be completely symmetrical : a model of the
impaired channel is connected to an inverse model of the
substitutive channel. Such an ideal system, has still to be
developed. Two of the presently available aids however follow
this symmetry principle, but only with a limited amount of
modelling. In the Tactile Vision Substitution System
(Bach-y-Rita et al., 1969) the video signal supplied by a
television camera is converted into mechanical or electrical
stimulation of the skin. The resolution of this system depends
on the number of elements in the stimulation matrix. The
connection between the two symmetrical parts of the prosthesis
is at the output of the transducer (A in Fig. 4). As the
visual signal has not been processed in the TVSS, it is not
committed to either of the two perceptual functions, and
depending on the choice of the matrix it can be used either in
pattern recognition tasks (Bach-y-Rita, 1972) or as a mobility
aid (Jansson, 1983). In the optophone (Fournier d'Albe, 1920)
and its more recent version the stereotoner (Smith, 1972), the
visual information is processed to a limited extend : the
inclination of the line segments of letters is translated into
pitch variations of sounds delivered to the auditory channel.
By the choice of the decoding parameter this system is
committed to text reading, a limited aspect of object
recognition. In this system the link between both symmetrical
parts of the prosthesis is at the level of the decoder (B in
Fig. 4). A special case seems to be the binaural sensory aid,
BSA, (Kay, 1974), in which the initial stages do not process
visual information. In the BSA, space is probed by a beam of
ultrasounds. The reflected ultrasounds are detected by two
receivers and converted to sounds delivered separately to the
ears. The distance of the obstacles is coded by the pitch of
the sounds delivered to the auditory system and their direction
by the binaural balance of sound intensity. Due to this
choices, this aid is committed to spatial localization. Six
sessions of 1 hour training are sufficient for blind persons to
demonstrate significant improvement in distance and direction
judgements (Wanet and Veraart, 1984). Because of the similarity
in functioning of the sensory substitution systems and the
sensory channels, it is likely that learning will be easier

254

with these systems than with completely artificial systems. Although only little testing has been done (Strelow, 1983), it seems thus likely that sensory substitution systems will be readily accepted by infants. Since the information has to be processed by a natural sensory channel in order to reach the perceptual level, sensorimotor interactions of the subject with this information will be maximized. One could even speculate that, although originally the visual character will be attributed to the substitutive information at the level of the amodal perceptual system, with further practice, a down regulation within the substitutive channel will make available this visual significance at a more peripheral level enhancing the possible sensorimotor interactions.

In conclusion, sensory substitution systems seem potentially the most interesting aids for blind persons : they are non-invasive, process information on-line, allow sensorimotor interaction with the environment and because of their similarity to the natural sensory channels require minimal training. To optimize their design one should model as closely as possible the two concerned sensory channels. The further this modelling is taken, the more one should distinguish between the two main functional roles of sensory channels : spatial localization and "object" recognition. With further technological developments one can hope to incorporate both functions into one prosthesis.

Acknowledgments. Part of this work was supported by a grant from the "Ministère de la Communauté française, Affaires sociales".

REFERENCES

Bach-y-Rita P. (1972) Brain Mechanisms in Sensory Substitution. Academic Press, New York & London.
Bach-y-Rita P., Collins C.C., Saunders F., White R. and Scadden L. (1969) Vision substitution by tactile image projection. Nature, 221 : 963-964.
Brindley G.S. and Lewin W.S. (1968) The sensations produced by electrical stimulation of the visual cortex. J. Physiol. (Lond.), 196 : 479-493.
Dobelle W.H., Quest D.O., Antunes J.L., Roberts T.S. and Girvin J.P. (1979) Artificial vision for the blind by electrical stimulation of the visual cortex. Neurosurgery, 5 : 521-527.
Fournier d'Albe E.E. (1920) The Optophone : An instrument for reading by ear. Nature, 105 : 295-296.
Jansson G. (1983) Tactile guidance of movement. Int. J. Neurosci. 19 : 37-46.
Kaas J.H., Merzenich M.M. and Killackey H.P. (1983) The reorganization of somatosensory cortex following peripheral nerve damage in adult and developing mammals. Ann. Rev. Neurosci. 6 : 325-356.
Kay L. (1974) A sonar aid to enhance spatial perception of the blind : engineering, design and evaluation. The Radio and Electronic engineer, 44 : 605-627.

Livingstone M.S. and Hubel D.H. (1983) Specificity of cortico-cortical connections in monkey visual system. Nature, 304 : 531-533.

Macko K.A., Jarvis C.D., Kennedy C., Miyaoka M., Shinohara M., Sokoloff L. and Mishkin M. (1982) Mapping the primate visual system with |2-^{14}|deoxyglucose. Science, 218 : 394-396.

Marr D. (1982) Vision. A computational Investigation into the Human Representation and Processing of Visual Information. W.H. Freeman and Company, San Francisco.

Nye P.W. and Bliss J.C. (1970) Sensory aids for the blind : a challenging problem with lessons for the future. Proceeding of the IEEE, 58 : 1878-1898.

Orban G.A. (1984) Neuronal operations in the visual cortex. Studies of Brain Function. Vol. 11. H.B. Barlow, T.H. Bullock, E. Florey, O.J. Grüsser & A. Peters (Eds.). Springer-Verlag, Berlin, 367 p.

Richard I., Veraart C. and Wanet M.-C. (1983) Space perception by blind subjects using an ultrasonic echo-locating prosthesis. J. Physiol. (Lond.), 345 : 126P.

Smith G.C. The stereotoner : a new reading aid for the blind. Proc. 25th Ann. Conf. Engin. Med. Biol., Bal Harbour, Fla., October 1972, p. 157.

Strelow E.R. (1983) Use of the binaural sensory aid by young children. J. of visual impairment and blindness, 77 : 429-437.

Tachi S., Tanie K., Komoriya K. and Abe M. (1982) Electrocutaneous communication in seeing-eye robot (Meldog). IEEE Trans. Biomed. Eng. 29 : 607.

von Holst E. and Mittelstaedt H. (1950) Das Reafferenzprinzip (Wechselwirkungen zwischen Zentral-nervensystem und Peripherie). Naturwissenschaften, 37 : 464-476.

Wanet M.-C. and Veraart C. (1984) Improvements in space coding by blind people by means of a sensory substitution system. Behav. Brain Res., in press.

DISCUSSION

François (to Gill)

I would like to make a small comment on what you said about
starting with a small market and then expanding into other mar-
kets outside a country. This is quite normal and is related to
an engineering problem. When you design something you can never
avoid making errors or building weaknesses into the system. Now,
it's very prudent to start off with a small number of units not
too far away so that you can support them completely. It is prudent to expand the system into other countries once you have a
higher degree of reliability built into the system. I've seen
people go broke because they started off on too large a scale.

Gill

There is a very small market penetration. There are less than
ten thousand reading aids in use in the world and under 9 thousand electronic mobility aids. It sounds quite a good number
until one compares it to 44 million blind people in the world
today. So the market penetration is minuscule. It probably takes
2 million or more pounds for new basic reading aids for the blind
to be evaluated and got in production. This is an enormous sum
of money when the market in your country may be very small. One
cannot justify the start of development unless you go to the international market in the end, because the development costs may
dominate the cost of the aid. One should consider if that money
would be better spent on building more lower technology devices,
simple electronic devices, costing 20 thousand pounds. Sighted
readers are extremely useful. If you look at it from just a cost
point of view, you takes an aid costing 23 thousand pounds, it
can last 5 years, and you spend 12% for annual maintenance. It
would be cheaper to have a sighted reader, even full time, eight
hours a day. It's not merely a financial calculation, it's one
that should be taken into account.

Question (to Graziani)

I have a few questions because I don't know if I understood you
correctly. Have you tried these pictures in embossed form or are
they just visual pictures, so far?

Graziani

I tried also a relief version of these images. Of course, as I
said before, only the simpler drawings can be perceived by touch.
When the drawings become complex, the control is difficult. But
they are drawings designed by myself. I know what they represent
and it's enough to control some characteristics. It's not important to perceive all the details. Only some things are perceived.
It's sufficient for the control.

Emiliani

In the second application presented, it's not a problem of producing images for the blind, but it's a problem of producing
images for sighted people. The blind produce drawings to communicate visual information to sighted people. Therefore, the
image can also be very complex. The blind can control if the
drawing they prepared is right, even if they do not perceive all
the details, but only some references in it.

Tobin

I'm wondering whether the computer experts can confirm that it
will be possible to do this. I'm thinking of the tactile graphical needs of blind children. During this study that I referred
to before, in the testing of mathematics, there were series of
bar graphs showing the number of children present in school each
day of the week. We are talking about 8 and 9 years old. What the
children would be asked to do, was to say on which day of the
week there were most children present and on which day of the
week there were fewer children present, or give specific numbers.
Now, when we put them into a tactile form, we found that the
blind children were not doing at all well on this. I think that
it was because a) there wasn't enough redundancy in the system,
and b) we are not taking account of the fact that the sense of
touch is not good at recognizing shapes but it is excellent at
recognizing texture differences. What was happening was that sometimes the children turned the page through 30° quite accidentally,
and the child would then say that, for example, one of the shorter bars was longer than another bar, because of its slope and its
orientation. The sense of touch wasn't good at recognizing that
difference. Will it be possible, using computers, to build in,
for example, textural differences which I'm going to represent at
the moment by lines, but which could of course also be represented
by the different intensities of dots, so that not only would the
child have available the opportunity to feel the shape, but would
also know that he was on another shape, because there was a textural difference as well? Would it be possible, using computer
graphics, to provide textural differences which are optimal for
the sense of touch, which would then also be valuable for a sighted reader because you can have these textural differences indicated by colours? You will be retaining the shape and size differences which would be valuable for his teacher and his sighted
colleagues, particularly in integrated settings. But we will be
increasing the probability of the child making correct deductions
because we are building in differences on more than one dimension.
Is this going to be possible? Are we going to get this into the
schools? I was administering a tactile intelligence test to blind
children which was very much a case of their recognizing perhaps
very slight changes in direction, and many of them were unable to

detect that the line had changed. If, of course, there was a
different texture available when it changed direction, then presumably we would increase the probability of them being able to
cope. Is this on?

Gill

The answer is "yes". The computer can produce quite a range of
textures in this sort of things, but it needs a human to specify
what it is to be coded and how. The human is essential to introduce extra information in the background information that the
computer could not interpret. Then, the computer can produce the
texture, the difference, all this sort of things, but the human
is essential to specify which is the optimum texture to use.
Then, you have the technical problems of producing the microtex-
ture, but technology is changing quite fast.

Jansson

This is a very interesting problem but, unfortunately, it is far
from solved. There are several people who have tried to get
discriminable textures with the aid of computers, but you can't
get a very large group. It's strange because, as you said, we know
that the fingers are very good at discriminating textures, but
we can't get them to work well with these plastic sheets. I think
there is a basic problem in the fact that we use the same material
for all the textures. There is some microstructure which masks
very much of the macrostructure we get into it. So, if we can get
different microstructures with the aid of the computer, we may
possibly solve the problem, but so far there have not been found
groups of more than 5-6-7 textures.

Thomsen

I think that the interesting thing about these bar graphs, whether
they are in a tactile form or in visual form, is what you can read
from them. Space recognition is very difficult for the blind, and
I think that our purpose and our aim should be to find the simplest
solution, and the simplest solution to this problem is to write
out a table with the numbers represented by the bars. I say that
because we could spend a lot of time and man power to find out the
solutions, how we could represent this in a tactile form. But
there is another and simpler solution to this, and I think to a
lot of other graphical problems, that you can write out the same
things in a more suitable form for the blind, so that the blind
will have access to exactly the same information.

Tobin

But, for example, in an integrated setting, when the teacher is
writing on the blackboard a triangle, it would be useful if the
blind child could feel the triangle and if the triangle could be
identified also with a different texture.

Warburg (to Powell)

Can this sort of schemes differentiate between low contrast situations as well as high contrast, and also could you program into the thing to recognize specific patterns - and I'm of course thinking of the human face?

Powell

In answer to the first question: the contrast sensitivity of the camera can be increased or the parameters of the computer algorithm may be changed to achieve greater sensitivity. In answer to the second question: it is the great advantage of computers over dedicated electronics that the program used can be changed rapidly. One program might be optimized for the recognition of a geographical landscape, another for reading a text, and yet another for recognizing faces.

Orban

This may be a very peripheral point, but I think it is a nice illustration of how long it takes in multidisciplinary workshops or conferences, and in all multidisciplinary efforts in general for changes in one discipline to be known by the other disciplines. You mentioned that the peripheral retina is probably specialized for motion perception and the central retina for form perception. I would very strongly dispute that view. Motion perception also is most refined in the center of the visual field, and the changes with eccentricity of those two functions, motion perception and form perception, are very different.

Powell

The issue I was concerned with here was the great disadvantage that a person with loss of peripheral vision has to suffer. Such a person is unable to sense potentially dangerous objects that are moving towards him if these objects fall outside the narrow angle of his central vision.

Werner

I am just curious about the algorithm for moving the center of your circles in order to detect curves and edges. Usually, you will probably scan a picture by running parallel to one direction first, then moving up and down. Is there any specific strategy?

Powell

I had envisaged that the person using a system such as this would move the camera in much the same way as one might hold a torch. In the demonstration I have simulated the position of the central focus that the user might employ to study a scene.

Question (to Powell)

I have a question as to the problem we all have to face. How do
you make a distinction between matter and light? The retinal image is built up from the reflection of objects, and we still can
recognize when we see an object or when we see a shadow, for example. May be, there is a special program to tell the brain
what's the object and what's the shadow. If we change the direction of the light it still can recognize objects. It rotates, but
it's still the same object. Did you put some of this in your
analysis for dealing with that problem? How can you tell what is
an object and what isn't? Is there some direction taken by you
to get to the problem?

Powell

Logical programming as exemplified by the language Prolog may be
valuable in answering this type of problem. Consider for example
the recognition of a teacup. A definition of a teacup might be:
a cylinder with solid sides, one end open, the other closed, a
semicircle (the handle) is attached to the outer face parallel
to the major axis of the cylinder. This specific definition if
combined with more general rules: a cylinder viewed along its
axis appears as a circle, a cylinder viewed at right angles to
its axis appears as a rectangle, etc., may enable an object to be
recognized in a variety of orientations. However, this type of
problem is not simple and I cannot claim it as a speciality.

Session 5: MOBILITY

Chairman: G. Bruun

Mobility Aids, Proposal for Research and Development
G. Bruun

Ergonomics, Mechanics and Functional Aspects of the
Long Cane
J. Walraven

The Role of Evaluation and of Inspiration in the
Development of Electronic Travel Aids for the Blind
A.D. Heyes

Development and Evaluation of Mobility Aids for the
Visually Handicapped
G. Jansson

Discussion

MOBILITY AIDS, PROPOSAL FOR RESEARCH AND DEVELOPMENT

G. Bruun
Electronics Laboratory, Electronics Institute,
Technical University of Denmark, Bldg. 344, 2800 Lyngby, Denmark

Mobility has been defined by Foulke (and cited in Brabyn 1982) as "the ability to travel safely, comfortably, gracefully and independently through the environment".

Electronic mobility aids have until now mainly been used as supplements to the long cane or the dog guide.

In order to have some reference for the following proposals for further possible developments we will briefly discuss examples of 3 types of mobility aids. All of them have obtained acceptance in several countries.

HAND-HELD SENSORS

The first type of aid to be considered is the hand-held sensor. Examples are the Mowat Sonar Sensor 1), shown Fig. 1, and the Nottingham Obstacle Detector 2).

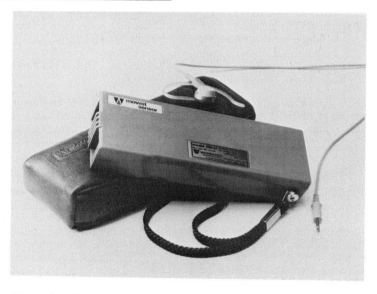

Fig. 1. Mowat Sonar Sensor.
(Wormald International Sensory Aids)

1) Developed in New Zealand by G.C. Mowat, manufactured by Wormald International Sensory Aids.

2) Blind Mobility Research Unit, Psychology Department, University of Nottingham, Nottingham, England.

The Mowat Sonar Sensor is used by a person using long cane or dog guide. He can for example use it to locate landmarks on his way (bus stop signs, doorways etc.). The sensor is a pulsed sonar which operates with an ultrasonic pulsed cone which is 15° wide and 30° high. It indicates the distance by vibrations with a frequency inversely proportional to the distance to the object detected. The range can be selected between maximal distances of 1 m and 3 m.

The Nottingham Obstacle Detector is a similar device. The operation frequency is 40 kHz. As an auditory readout a loudspeaker or an earphone is provided. The range, which is 2.10 m is subdivided into intervals of 30 cm. To each interval there is a corresponding note of the major musical scale. The tone signal goes down the scale as one approaches the target.

Both two sensors have the limitation that they can only sense in one direction at a time. In order to obtain spacial information one will have to move the ray in two directions. A person experienced in its use can, however, have good use of the instrument. This holds particularly for cases when he needs orientation that cannot be obtained by means of the long cane.

Proposal for further development:

o In order to obtain improved resolution in the distance-
   indication, the sensor might be provided with a line of
   closely located vibrating points to be sensed by the tip
   of a finger. This addition might be of help in situations
   when more than one reflection occurs at a time.

o Some experiments with various shapes of the ultrasonic
   beam might also be of use.

An electronic device of the kind mentioned should be so simple to use that most blind persons should have one - if not for any other reason - to obtain better perception of indoor localities.

SONICGUIDE

The Sonicguide [1] represents a type of aid by means of which the user can be informed about obstacles located in a horizontal plane in front of the persons head. Fig. 2 shows how the device is incorporated into an eyeglass frame. An ultrasound frequency-modulated signal is transmitted from a transducer mounted in the center of the eyeglass. The beam is directed straight ahead. Two receivers are directed 15° to the left and right of the transmitter beam. The received signals are dealt with separately as they are multiplied by the transmitted signal and the resulting low-frequency difference signals are led to the respective ears through tubes which do not obstruct ambient sound. The FM-radar system employed is illustrated in Fig. 3.

1) Developed by Kay at the University of Canterbury, Christchurch, New Zealand. It is manufactured by Wormald International Sensory Aids Ltd., Christchurch.
   Distributer: Telesensory System Inc.

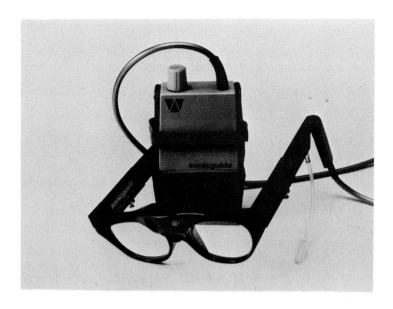

Fig. 2. Sonicguide.
(Wormald International Sensory Aids)

The user is able to judge the distance to a reflecting object from the pitch of the sound. The direction is obtained from a judgment of the relative loudness of the particular sound to the two ears.

The timbre of the signal gives information about the type of reflection, e.g. whether the surface is rough or smooth. Echoes from leaves will for example give multi-component reflections to be recognized by the experienced user.

The vertical range of the device is limited to about knee-hight, and the user has to rely upon his long cane when detecting curbs.

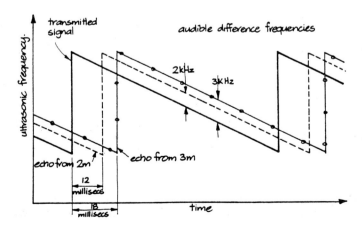

Fig. 3. The FM-radar-principle of the Sonicguide
(Sonicguide Handbook)

The Sonicguide gives a lot of information to digest by its user. Therefore it takes many hours to learn. An intensive course could for example take 30 hours a week for 4 weeks. From the information available from the device, however, the proficient user can obtain a varied impression of his surroundings. Further, he will be able to avoid obstacles at head-hight and he will be warned by many obstacles before being warned by the long cane.

For children a special kind of Sonicguide: Canterbury Child's Aid, see Strelow et al. 1978 and Boys et al. 1979. This device is mounted on a headband, rather than eyeglasses. One of the main differences betwwen this aid and the Sonicguide is that the childrens aid has a shorter range which is most relevant to children for example when they are at play.

Some of the problems or limitations of the Sonicguide are the following:

- Doppler-effect causes error in the determination of distance when an obstacle moves towards or away from the device. Objects approaching (or being approached) will be sensed as being further away than in reality.

  An example taken from the instruction book is as follows: A person walking at a rapid pace of 1.5 m per second towards a wall will hear an upward shift in frequency of 1300 Hz. The result is that when he is 2 m from the wall, he will perceive the distance to be 3.5 m. This effect is of course important to take into account during training.

- Users who are born blind are often very good at using the natural accoustic reflections when walking through a crowded area. They will therefore be hesitant about using a device if it takes so much of their audio-attention that they have a hard time using their natural accoustic orientation. Persons who appreciate the Sonicguide will therefore more often be found among late-blind users. It should, however, be pointed out once more, that the Sonicguide allows for ambient hearing as the tubes leading to the ears will normally be open.

- Some users tend to avoid any electronic aid. Using the Sonicguide means not only wearing special eyeglasses, but also taking care of the connection by wire to the instrument box and making sure the battery is charged.

- Some users claim that they find it difficult to know when the battery needs charging.

Sonicguide teachers estimate[1] the number of potential Sonicguide users in Denmark (pop. 5.1 M) to be about 2% of the total blind population which is about 15000. This amounts to 300 potential users, which is about 10% of those who are totally blind.

Before completing this section: it is fascinating to see a Sonicguide-user with long cane walking fast on the sidewalk of

_____
1) See Østergaard et al. 1980, p. 23.

a busy street avoiding collisions and without having to touch
hindrances with the cane.

Sonicguide: Proposal for further development.

Some problems for research and development related to or inspired by the Sonicguide are the following:

o   how could curb-detection be incorporated into a system
    like the Sonicguide?

    Perhaps by combination of the present system and a laser
    device as used in the Laser Cane,

o   is the Doppler-problem something the user should be able
    to accept, or should one try to get rid of the problem.
    When the FM-signal has an increasing frequency slope (oppo-
    site to the situation in Fig. 3) the Doppler-effect will
    cause an error which is opposite to the one discussed a-
    bove. Therefore one could make a system which detects the
    relative motion of the object. In this system the frequen-
    cy should have a rising and falling slope in alternate pe-
    riods of the modulating signal. Or one could - in order to
    be able to detect if the object is approaching or leaving
    - use a rising frequency in one period and a decreasing
    frequency in the next two periods of the modulating signal,

o   a simple means for users to determine the remaining bat-
    tery-life-time, ought to be developed. (By the way: life-
    time determination is also a problem with the small bat-
    teries used in hearing aids),

o   the ability of the Sonicguide to operate at changing tem-
    peratures and at high humidity (rain) ought to be investi-
    gated and - if necessary - improved,

o   other types of possible displays could be investigated.
    A vibrating display to be mounted some discrete place on
    the skin might be of interest.

    It could for example consist of two lines of small vibra-
    tors mounted on the upper-arms.

    Using such tactile displays the Sonicguide system might
    have to be changed from an FM-system to a pulsed system,
    or the FM-system would have to be decoded to obtain direct
    spacial information. Such a decoding is used in normal FM-
    radars.

o   Socio-psychological studies should be made, for example re-
    lated to the teaching situation. They could help finding
    out how to make prospective devices most acceptable to the
    users.

LASER CANES

The Laser Cane is a long cane provided with a number - for example 4 - gallium-arsenide injection lasers which emit short
(0.2 µS) pulses of infrared light (9050 Ångström). The repeti-

tion frequency is low (40-80 Hz). The lasers are directed such
that the beams are within the semi-plane which corresponds to
the direction of walk. Light from the reflection of the narrow
beams is detected by directive photosensitive receivers. Because of the narrow beams and also the relatively narrow angles
within which the receivers detect, the system can determine the
distance to an obstacle by triangulation. The principle of the
C5 Laser Cane (Farmer 1980) is shown in Fig. 4.

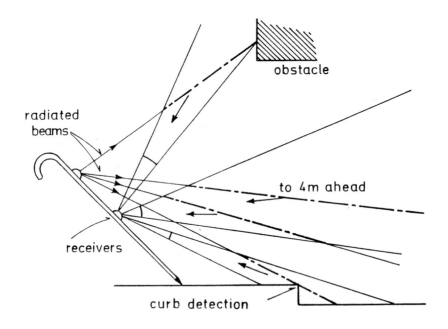

Fig. 4. Laser Cane principle

In case an obstacle is detected by one of the three upper beams,
the blind user will hear a sound in an earphone or sense a vibration by his index finger.

Another signal warns the user when - in case of a downstep -
the lower beam fails to be detected.

In the design of a Laser Cane there is a question as to how
much information should be provided to the blind user. In the
development of the Swedish Laser Cane (Fornaus & Jansson 1975)
the emphasis has been to make a simple, inexpensive, light
weight aid. The instrument has only one channel as it was assumed that the user could not utilize the information from a
3-channel device. In Farmer 1982 it is, however, pointed out,
that this belief is contradicted by the experience with the
American Bionic Laser Cane.

LIMITATIONS AND PROBLEMS WITH THE LASER CANE

Some of the problems related to the use of the Laser Cane are:
- it does not receive reflections from clear glass plate,
- in its present form, low objects cannot be detected,
- it tends to fail when snowing,
- the user has trouble with directing the cane pointed in the direction of walk.

Laser Cane: Proposal for further research and development.

Some of the problems to be investigated are similar to those related to the Sonicguide. Only two problems, which are related, will be mentioned:

o the user might obtain a more detailed information about the obstacles in front of him if more lasers and detectors were employed. In such a system - in order to make the presentation acceptable - a relatively sophisticated signal processing might be needed,

o in case of a device like the one mentioned above one might need a tactile display like the type discussed in connection with the Sonicguide.

POSSIBLE MOBILITY AIDS FOR THE FUTURE

The paper by Brabyn (1982) discusses various ideas for instruments some of which might lead to useable mobility aids in the future. In such devices information can for example be picked up by TV-cameras or by refined ultrasound transducer arrays. In most cases the main problem seems to be the presentation of the information available in a way such that it can be utilized by the blind user.

Some of the problems:
o to extract information from a stereoscopic system of TV-cameras about directions and distances to objects,

o to study how such information can be reduced to a particular level suitable for the user,

o to study various forms of displays, for example consisting of matrixes of vibrators,

o to study learning curves related to various levels of information displayed.

If one uses a system of ultrasound transducers in a phased array, information about distances and directions can - at least in principle - easily be found. A problem related to such a system could be:

o should one concentrate one a 2 or 3 dimensional system. In the paper by Brabyn 1982 a system with a PPI-type of display is referred to (Brabyn et al. 1981).

In the above discussion most emphasis has been put upon tactile displays. Even if in many situations one wants to use the ear only for listening to ambient sounds, one should recognize the great ability for signal handling of the hearing system. Therefore future studies should also deal with audio displays.

To-day various forms of audio displays play a role in mobility aids. Auditory codes have also been used in reading aids for the blind. In a paper by Fish 1976 one particular code is investigated experimentally. Using this code two-dimensional pictures can be displayed. A dot in the picture is represented by a tone burst, the frequency of which represents the one dimension, whereas the other dimension is represented by the ratio of sound amplitudes to the two ears.

o Extensive evaluations of other auditory codes ought to be performed.

   In particular there seems to be a need for codes for monoaural representation.

CONCLUSION

From the preceeding discussions it can be concluded that research and development within the field of mobility aids should deal with:

- the main principles to be used in the aids
- development and evaluation of displays

Related to tactile displays, there is a great need for looking into problems related to the physiology of the user. In addition there are many practical matters related to electromechanical design and to optimizing the design for low power consumption.

ACKNOWLEDGEMENT

The author wishes to thank Erik Østergaard, mobility teacher at the Institute for the Blind, Copenhagen, for helpful information about mobility aids and experience from mobility courses.

REFERENCES

John A. Brabyn, "New developments in mobility and orientation aids for the blind", IEEE Trans. on Biomedical Eng., BME-29, April 1982, pp. 285-289.

J.A. Brabyn, C.C. Collins and L. Kay, "A wide bandwidth CTFM scanning sonar with tactile and acoustic display for persons with impaired vision (blind, diver, etc.)", Proc. Ultrason. Int. Conf., Brighton, England, July 2, 1981.

J.T. Boys, E.R. Strelow and G.R.S. Clark, "A prosthetic aid for a developing blind child", Ultrasonics, Jan.1979,pp.37-42.

Leicester W. Farmer, "Mobility devices, pp. 357-412, in: Foundations of Orientation and Mobility ed. R.L. Welsh & B.B. Blasch, American Foundation for the Blind, N.Y.1980. (This paper contains a bibliography).

Raymond M. Fish, "An audio display for the blind", IEEE Trans. on Biomedical Eng., BME-23, March 1976, pp. 144-154.

L. Fornaus, D.G. Jansson, "The Swedish Laser Cane-development and evaluation", Report on European Conference on Technical Aids for the Visually Handicapped, Stockholm, Handikappinstitutet, August 1974, pp. 61-65.

L. Kay, "An ultrasonic sensing probe as a mobility aid for the Blind", Ultrasonics, April-June 1964, pp. 53-59.

E.R. Strelow, N. Kay and L. Kay, "Binanural Sensory Aid: Case studies of its use by two children", Journ. Visual Impairment and Blindness, Jan. 1978, pp. 1-9.

S. Tachi, R.W. Mann and D. Rowell, "Quantitative comparison of alternative sensory displays for mobility aids for the Blind", IEEE Trans. on Biomedical Eng., BME-30, Sept.1983, pp. 571-577.

E. Østergaard, V. Transe Rasmussen, G. Bjerre and W. Williams, "Report on work with Sonicguide", Institute for the Blind, Copenhagen 1980, (in Danish).

ERGONOMICS, MECHANICS AND FUNCTIONAL ASPECTS OF THE LONG CANE

J. Walraven
Institute for Perception TNO
Kampweg 5,
3769 ZG Soesterberg, The Netherlands

INTRODUCTION

In spite of all the effort put into the development of electronic mobility aids, we still have a long way to go before we can offer the visually handicapped a device that can fully replace the (long) cane (e.g. Jansson, 1975; Armstrong, 1977). Therefore, this indispensible aid deserves the full attention of the rehabilitation engineer, and the more so because it seems so deceptively easy to manufacture. As Thornton (1977) already remarked: "In spite of all experimentation, the ideal cane which meets all the requirements has yet to be found". This conclusion is as valid today, as it was seven years ago.

Actually it is very hard to define the "ideal" cane. The point is, that the cane has to meet different, often conflicting, demands. For example, it is difficult to make a cane that is both collapsible and as strong and dependable as a rigid cane. This is probably one of the main problems in modern cane design and, unfortunately, one which has not always been recognised. Right now therefore, there are quite a few canes about that are not fully equal to their task. It was for that reason that our Institute was asked by the Stichting Warenonderzoek Gehandicapten (SWOG), a recently founded Dutch consumer organisation for the handicapped, to make a study of this field, and develop criteria for separating the good from the bad canes (Walraven, 1982).

As a first step in that direction we collected the assortment of canes available in the Netherlands at that time. We subjected these to a thorough ergonomical analysis, hereby guided by the experience obtained from interviews with users and the information obtained from a literature survey. We also did some measurements for evaluating functional aspects, but these were of a very preliminary nature, meant only to demonstrate the feasibility of getting more objective criteria for cane evaluation.

In the following we shall discuss what we have learnt from that study, and how that may be put to use for the design of better canes.

THE TEST SAMPLE

The different canes tested, eight in total, fall into two categories: rigid and collapsible. The latter category includes both folding and telescopic canes (see Fig.1). Note, however, that some of these canes cannot be fully collapsed, and thus are not very effective as such.

The canes, which have been numbered from 1-8, show large differences in design. Their main characteristics can be summarised as follows:
no. 1. A rigid cane made of solid fibreglass. The (tapering)shaft is light and flexible.
no. 2. A rigid, tubular cane, also made of fibreglass. The cane is rather short (1 m) possibly because it is mainly intended for signalling. This (Japanese) cane is equipped with a pulsing red light (LED) inserted in the hollow of the shaft.

276

no. 3. Two-section folding cane of tubular aluminium, held together by an elastic tie.
no. 4. Four-section folding cane of tubular aluminium, held together by a plastic-coated steel cable (Hycor cane).
no. 5. Five-section folding cane of plastic-coated tubular brass, held together by an elastic tie.
no. 6. Two-section telescopic cane of tubular aluminium with crook handle. The two sections are connected by an internal expansion joint.
no. 7. Three-section telescopic cane of tubular aluminium with crook handle. Similar locking principle as used for cane 6. This cane can also be used as a means of support.
no. 8. Five-section telescopic cane made of fibreglass. The tapering sections are "locked" by friction between inner and outer surfaces of adjoining sections.

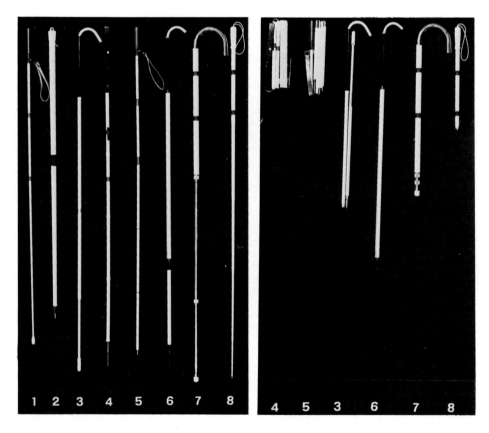

Figure 1. The various canes tested in this study (left). The non-rigid canes of this sample are also shown in the collapsed state (right).

This is, of course, a relatively small sample of the great variety of canes produced all over the world. It will do, however, for illustrating the main principles of current cane design.

ERGONOMICS AND MECHANICS OF THE CANE

A cane can be functionally divided into three components.
- the grip
- the shaft (either rigid or none-rigid)
- the tip

Each of these elements may have to meet quite different demands when the cane is not only used as a probing instrument, but also as a means of support. Here we shall not go into this problem however, and focus only on its function as an obstacle detector. In doing so we shall not always detail the arguments and criteria underlying our evaluation. Most of these are based on common sense anyway, rahter than on profound theoretical foundations.

The grip

The main points we want to make with respect to the grip can be summarised as follows
- the grip should be easily replaceable
- non-slippery
- sweat resistant
- non-fraying
- of sufficient length to allow some shifting of the hand position (for balance)
- have a provision for attachment to the wrist (or for suspending the cane) like a crook or (adjustable) wrist loop.

In our sample of canes there actually was no cane that met all the requirements. There was one (no.3), equipped with a golf grip and crook, that seemed quite adequate, although replacing the golfgrip poses a problem.

There are also canes without any grip at all (nos. 2 and 8), which in case of a fibreglass cane may be preferable to a badly designed grip.

The shaft

The shaft is the main determinant of the cane's performance. Important in this respect are the material employed and the construction (rigid or non-rigid).

Modern canes are made of either aluminium or fibreglass. We would prefer a good quality fibreglass, because this material is more flexible, and hence, less prone to deformation. One should realise in this respect, that canes can be subjected to quite strong transversal forces. This may happen for example, when the cane gets stuck at the "backhand" side of the user, causing him to trip over his own cane. Solid fibreglass may provide for a virtually indestructible cane, but such canes are not produced in collapsible form. Most cane users prefer a non-rigid cane, and for good reasons. When not walking, the cane becomes a useless appendage and a nuisance (particularly in a crowded bus or train); it also occupies one hand. Furthermore, a blind person does not want always to advertise his handicap.

The non-rigid canes are generally of two kinds, telescopic or folding, each with their specific (dis)advantages.

The telescope construction

The telescoping principle has two distinct advantages: it can be made relatively rigid, and can also be very compact. The compactness can only be achieved, however, if all sections have about the same length, the largest one determining the size of the cane in the collapsed state. Taking 25 cm as an upper limit, this means that one needs 5-6 sections for covering the normal range of cane lengths. This also means that the cane has about as many joints, all of which have to be separately locked and unlocked. There are canes which simply have no locks at all, hereby relying on friction between the (tapering) sections (as in cane no.5). This attractive principle is illustrated in Fig.2.

Unfortunately, the friction force that keeps the segments in place is not always strong enough to resist the axially directed forces that may result upon hitting an obstruction. This means that one must be prepared to regularly refasten the loosened sections. Right now we are in the process of developing a new type of locking device for this kind of cane, but we

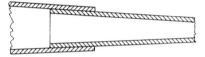

Figure 2. Tapering joints of a telescope cane without locking mechanism.

too have not yet been able to overcome all technical problems.

The other types of telescopic canes that are currently available are equipped with expansion locks, which are fastened or loosened by twisting the sections. There usually are only two or three sections, which means that the advantage of compactness is lost, Therefore, we believe that only the principle shown in Fig.2 is suited for telescopic canes (provided an adequate locking device is developed). Otherwise, the folding cane seems to be a more promising candidate for the "ideal" collapsible cane.

The folding construction

The folding construction of commercially available canes invariably consists of joined sections of hollow aluminium or fibreglass, held together by a tension member. The cane joints may be straight, flared, or both. Straight joints (see Fig. 3a) offer greater rigidity, but are prone to wear due to burring of the edge. This damage to the edges in combination with the close fit of male and female segments (as is required for ensuring good connectivity), may also seriously hamper the assemblance of the cane. Flared joints do not have this problem, since they are always self-aligning (see Fig. 3b), even after being subjected to considerable wear. However, their resistance to lateral displacement is much less than that of straight joints, and they may also tend to jam. The best solution therefore, is a combination of flared and straight joint as illustrated in Fig.3c. For a more detailed account of joint principles and their mechanical consequences, see Grossman and Judd (1977).

There are more ways to construct a collapsible cane, of course. Some original attempts, like for example a telescopic cane with pneumatic locking of the joints, have been made at the Massachusetts Institute of Technology (Baumann et al., 1963). So far, however, only the telescopic and

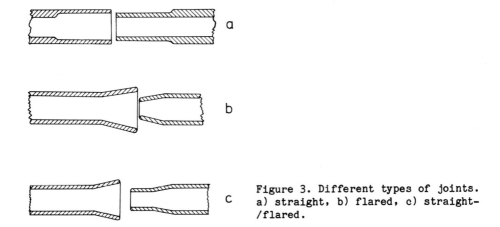

Figure 3. Different types of joints.
a) straight, b) flared, c) straight-
/flared.

the folding mechanism described here, have found acceptance, probably because these principles provide the best solution in terms of reliability and cost-effectiveness.

One of the main factors determining the reliability of the folding cane is the durability of the tension member. Elastic cords are subject to wear because they get stretched over the edges of the joints (when the cane is folded). These edges should be blunted of beveled, therefore, and the cord be sheeted in some kind of protective tubing, preferably polypropylene of nylon.

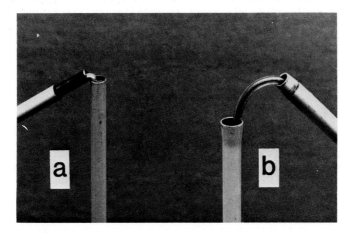

Figure 4. Elastic tie (a) and plastic-sheated steel cable (b). The former
is stretched tautly over the edge of the joint, and therefore,
has a very short life-span.

The problem of breaking of the elastic tie can be avoided by using a nylon cord or steel cable instead (See Fig.4). The latter are slackened when the cane is collapsed, and thus less vulnerable to damage by the sharp edges of the joints. The construction of the cane may become a little more complicated however, due to the need for a tensing device.

On the basis of the considerations discussed above we have come to the conclusion that both the telescopic and folding principle are suitable candidates for constructing a non-rigid cane. The former provides the smallest package when collapsed, but poses an engineering problem (locking mechanism) which has not been resolved as yet. Right now, therefore, the folding principle seems to be the most sensible choice for constructing a collapsible cane. The latter should preferably posses the following features

- joints of the straight/flared type (Fig. 3c)
- a shaft made of high quality fibreglass
- a durable and easily replaceable tension member

As for the latter requirement this might be met by employing a nylon cord or steel cable rather than an elastic tension member.

The tip

The tip of the cane is usually made of nylon or (nickel-plated) steel. Steel has been claimed to provide for a somewhat better acoustical and tactile performance of the cane (see later). On the other hand, the nylon tip is less heavy and thus provides for a better balance. Irrespective of the choice of material, one should always strive for

- easy replacement (for example a screw-on tip)
- smooth transition from cane to tip (to prevent that the tip gets stuck)
- durability, which implies sufficient length in the case of a nylon tip

As already mentioned above, the question whether a nylon or steel tip should be used, is often discussed in relation to the transfer of tactile and/or acoustic information. This issue will be addressed in the next section, in which we shall touch on the various functional aspects of the cane.

FUNCTIONAL ASPECTS

The main function of the long cane is to provide both tactile and acoustic information about obstacles, and also, about changes in the texture of the pavement (guide function). In addition, the cane has a signaling function identifying its user as being visually handicapped. In the following we shall discuss these functions, and their possible consequences for cane design, in more detail.

Tactile information transfer

Tapping or scratching the ground with a cane produces vibrations, that may convey information about the surface in question. Ungar (1978) recorded surface-specific vibration spectra transferred by the cane, as measured by three tiny (2 g) accelerometers (one for each spatial direction), attached to the cane shaft. He was thus able to show differences in discrimination performance of rigid and non-rigid canes. However, he did not investigate whether these physically measured differences were relevant, that is, correlated with human performance data.

A more direct approach for evaluating the vibro-tactile discriminatory performance of a cane, is to test how well subjects can identify a variety of, for example, pavement-surface textures. This has recently been investigated in a study by Schenkman (1983a). He found no significant differences between canes when comparing discrimination performance for four different pavement surfaces, i.e. concrete, linoleum, (moist) sand, and asphalt. The subjects were instructed to tap only, however. According to Schenkman, differences between canes would probably have been found if the subjects had also been allowed to make scraping movements.

In the absence of any other data showing vibratory discrimination to be critically dependent on cane parameters, it is not possible as yet, to assess the importance of this aspect in relation to cane design. One may expect, however, that the lighter and the more rigid the cane, the better its vibration transfer.

Acoustic information transfer

The sound produced by the tap of a cane is received both directly and indirectly (i.e. after reflection). The indirect component is of particular importance with respect to echo-location (e.g. Cotzin and Dallenbach, 1950; Wilson, 1966). We shall now first consider however, the information conveyed by the directly received sound, both with respect to sound pressure level (loudness) and acoustic spectrum (tonality).

In Fig.5 data of Grossman and Judd (1977) are plotted, which show sound pressure levels recorded from 10 different canes, when tapping on tiles, wood or cement. It is of interest that the results obtained with nylon and metal tips respectively, show no systematic differences.

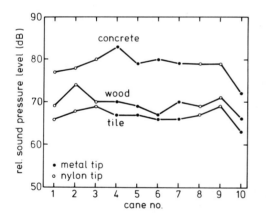

Figure 5. Sound pressure levels measured when tapping the cane on tiles, wood and cement, respectively. Results from 10 different canes, either with metal (•) or nylon (o) tip. Data from Grossman and Judd (1977).

Ungar (1978) measured the acoustic discrimination performance of 24 canes in terms of changes in the frequency spectrum of the tap. He found that some canes may indeed perform better than others in this respect. Fig.6 shows an example of his results, for a rigid cane with metal tip (no.17) and a non-rigid cane with nylon tip (no.3). In general, metal tips (and shafts) were found to provide better spectral discrimination. Unfortunately Ungar (1978) did not investigate whether these physical differences could be correlated with performance measures of acoustical discrimination.

In addition to the spectral characteristics one also has to consider the temporal waveform of the sound pulses produced by tapping the cane. This could be of relevance with respect to echo-location.

282

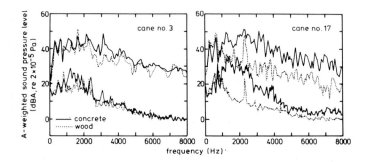

Figure 6. Frequency spectra of the sound produced by a non-rigid cane with nylon tip (left) and rigid cane with metal tip (right). The two upper traces show the result for tapping, either on wood or cement, whereas the two lower traces show the same for scraping. Data from Ungar (1978).

In order to see how canes might physically differ in this respect we made some recordings in the anechoic room of our laboratory. The taps were produced on a tile placed on a block of dense foam plastic. Tapping was done by hand, hereby watching the meter readings of the sound pressure meter (Brüel & Kjaer, type 2218) for maintaining a constant loudness level. The taps were also spectrally analysed (Hewlett & Packard, type 8064A), but these data did not discriminate very much between canes. They all showed similar frequency spectra with a rather flat optimum of 30-40 dB in the 2000-8000 Hz region.

Fig.7 shows the waveforms of the sound pulse produced by the various canes of our test assortment. It is clear that there are differences between canes. However, we do not know as yet, whether these differences are sufficient to discriminate between the various canes with regard to echo-location. There is evidence of a small echo in the recordings, which was probably produced by some nearby equipment in the room. It is most

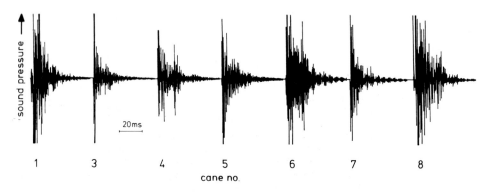

Figure 7. Waveform of the sound pulse produced by various canes.

distinct for canes 4 and 6, but it is almost absent (for reasons unknown) in canes 3 and 7. These are just preliminary results however, and we have not tried to correlate them with mechanical characteristics of the canes in question.

Schenkman (1983b) studied echo-location (under laboratory conditions), employing trained cane users as subjects. His carefully controlled experiments produced interesting results, but these do not allow, as yet, inferences with respect to what kind of cane properties are of particular importance for echo-location. His data provide some support, however, for the notion that a steel tip may be more effective in this respect than a nylon tip; at least, for objects located at distances in excess of about 4 m. At the shorter distances tested (1.70 m and 2.74 m) there were no significant differences in performance when using either a nylon or a steel tip. The advantage of the steel tip at larger distances is presumably due to the higher sound pressure level produced. However, steel tips do not necessarily produce always more sound than nylon tips (see Fig.5).

Summarising this section on the acoustic properties of the cane we conclude that although physical measures have been reported which show that canes may differ in their capability of acoustic discrimination and echo-location, the link with user performance measures is still rather weak. The few data that are available suggest that, as far as the acoustic identification of pavement or floor materials is concerned, rigidity of the cane has a positive effect on performance.

Probe function

To be useful as an obstacle detector, the cane must have a certain minimum length (for early warning). This length should be matched to the step length (Lazarus and Harrell, 1977), to enable putting one's foot at a place that has been cleared during the preceding sweep of the cane. Uslan (1978, 1980) published tables in which cane length is given as a function of both step length (37-63 cm) and height at which the cane is held above ground level (100-125 cm). We found that his data can be reasonably well fitted by the relation

$$L = S + 55 + 0.75 (H-100)$$

where L and S are cane and step length, respectively, and H is the height of the hand position (everything measured in cm).

However, the length of the cane may also depend on the particular way in which it is held, that is, with the hand in front of or at the side of the body. We would refrain, therefore, from giving strict rules, and rather let the user find empirically what length is best suited for him. It might be helpful in this respect if the grip could be adjusted in position or length. A simple solution would be to have a relatively long grip, so as to allow some freedom in positioning the hand.

A second point to pay attention to is the balance and weight of the cane. Most of the time the cane will be in the lifted position, in which it may exert a fairly substantial torque on the wrist, particarly when the cane is long and equipped with a heavy metal point. It would be advisable, therefore to have the centra of gravity as close to the wrist as possible. Preliminary results from an experiment by Shingledecker (1975) are consistent with this view. It might be worthwhile even, although this has not been systematically studied, to add some counter weight at the grip end of the cane, like for example, a heavy crook or knob. The well known Equipoise cane with its robust aluminium crook, might be taken as a point in case (Thornton, 1977).

Signal function

The white colour of the cane serves the purpose of identifying its user as visually handicapped, and also to make the cane more conspicuous. The latter function is of particular importance when the cane is used to signal one's intent to cross the street. The cane should be visible, then, at a distance sufficiently large to allow approaching vehicles to stop in time. If the latter approach at a speed of 50 km/h, one may estimate this recognition distance to be about 70 m (SWOV, 1970).

We did some pilot experiments (Walraven, 1983) in which we measured the distance at which the various canes of our assortment could still be recognised as such. The values we obtained ranged from 31 to 92 m, a variability caused by the differences in thicknesses of the canes and the materials used for coating them. Retro-reflecting coatings turned out to be less effective in this respect (in daylight). This was to be expected because they reflect most of the incident light in the direction of the light source, (the sky), and thus look less white in the day-time than a diffusely reflecting coating. It is still a subject of debate whether this disadvantage is outweighed by the better visibility of the cane at night. Perhaps it would be more sensible to improve the visibility of the diurnal cane traveller himself, by using, for example, reflectorised armlets.

CANE EVALUATION

On the basis of the expertise obtained in this study a checklist was made for evaluating the ergonomics, the mechanics, and the functional aspects of the long cane. Table I shows how our canes scored on this list. However, due to the limited scope of this study, not all entries have been completed. Thus there are no ratings of the acoustical and tactile performance of the canes. Neither did we obtain quantitative measures of mechanical characteristics for defining "rigidity" and "deformation resistance" of the cane.

Table I   Checklist for cane evaluation. Ratings are given on a five-point scale, that is: excellent (++), good (+), average (±), bad (-), very bad (--).

design features		cane number 1	2	3	4	5	6	7	8
grip	: comfort	±	0	+	±	±	+	0	±
	replaceability	--	0	-	+	++	++	0	-
	construction	-	0	±	-	-	+	0	-
crook	: effectiveness	0	0	+	0	0	±	+	0
	construction	0	0	±	0	0	+	±	0
shaft	: rigidity	--	+	±	+	-	+	++	-
	deformation resistance	++	++	±	±	-	±	±	+
	durability	++	++	+	±	±	+	±	-
folding	: compactness	0	0	±	+	+	0	0	0
mechanism	joints	0	0	++	±	--	0	0	0
	tension member	0	0	-	-	--	0	0	0
	replacement	0	0	-	-	±	0	0	0

Table I (Cont'd)

design features		cane number							
		1	2	3	4	5	6	7	8
telescope	: compactness	0	0	0	0	0	±	±	++
mechanism	locking mechanism	0	0	0	0	0	+	±	-
tip	: shape	+	++	++	++	+	±	+	-
	attachment	++	++	++	++	±	-	+	+
	durability	+	++	+	+	++	-	+	-
	replaceability	--	--	++	-	±	--	+	-
acoustic	: discrimination								
function	echo-location								
tactile	: discrimination								
function									
signal	: night	-	+	--	+	-	±	±	±
function	daytime	--	+	+	-	-	+	-	-
probe	: balance	++	+	+	+	-	-	-	++
function	weight	++	±	±	-	-	-	--	++
		++	-	+	±	-	+	+	-
overall quality rating		+	-	±	±	--	±	-	±

As Table I shows, none of the canes tested obtained a positive rating
on all check points. There was only one cane that might be considered to be
a good cane (no.1), but since it was a non-rigid one, it still would be
unacceptable for the majority of cane users. One of the canes in our
assortment (no.5) represents a prime example of poor design. It is a
folding cane made of heavy brass tubing connected by the worst kind of
straight joints. These repeatedly came loose because of the considerable
force required when disassembling jammed segments. Also, the edges of the
joints were not beveled and thus played havock with the (unprotected)
elastic tie (see Fig.4). The latter was at one end attached to the tip by
means of a socket clamp that had to be fitted by a special tool. Replacement of the tip was possible only by cutting the tie. The cane was badly
balanced, had a tendency to wiggle and put a heavy strain on the wrist. It
also happens to be the cane that, until recently, was sold best!

CONCLUSION

This study shows that it is apparently not that simple to design a collapsible cane that meets all the requirements. We fully agree with MacNeal
(1980) therefore, who concluded that the ideal collapsible cane provides a
real challenge to the rehabilition engineer. The conclusions and suggestions put forward here, most of which are actually not that original, might
serve as guide lines for attaining that goal.
    The fact that a poorly designed cane may nevertheless become a best-
seller, shows the need for (qualified) counseling organisations for the
visually handicapped. This is not sufficient however, because such organis-

ations can only aid in making the best choice among the available products. What we really need is more research to improve the quality of these products.

ACKNOWLEDGMENTS

This research was partly supported by the Stichting Warenonderzoek Gehandicapten (SWOG).

REFERENCES

Armstrong, J.D.(1977). Mobility aids and the limitations of technological solutions. New Beacon 61, 113-115.

Cotzin, M. and Dallenbach, K.M. (1950). Facial vision: the role of pitch and loudness in the perception of obstacles by the blind. Am.J.Psychol. 63, 485-515.

Grossman, P.J. and Judd, R.P. (1977). Mechanical evaluation of non-rigid canes. American Foundation for the Blind, New York.

Jansson, G. (1975). The detection of objects by the blind with the aid of a laser cane. Rep. 172, Dept. of Psychol. University of Uppsala.

Lazarus, R.S. and Harrell, B.B. (1977). A guideline and formula for determining proper cane length. Long Cane News 10, 22-30.

Schenkman, B.N. (1983a) Identification of ground materials with the aid of tapping sounds and vibrations of long canes for the blind. Uppsala Psychological Report No. 367. University of Uppsala, Department of Psychology.

Schenkman, B.N.(1983b) Human echolocation as a function of kind of sound source and object position. Uppsala Psychological Report no. 363. University of Uppsala, Department of Psychology.

Shingledecker, C.A. (1975). The development of an improved cane for the blind pedestrian. In: Annual Report by E. Foulke. Perceptual Alternatives Laboratory, University of Louisville.

SWOV (1970) Verkeerstekens op borden. Rapport 1970-7a, Stichting Wetenschappelijk Onderzoek Verkeersveiligheid, The Hague.

Thornton, W. (1977). Long canes. The New Beacon, Febr. '77, 39-40.

Ungar, E.E. (1978). Sound and vibration characterization of canes for the blind. American Foundation for the Blind, New York.

Uslan, M.M. (1978). Cane technique: Modifying the touch technique for full path coverage. J. of Visual Impairment and Blindness 72, 10-14.

Uslan, M.M. (1980). Drop-off detection in the touch technique. J. Visual Impairment and Blindness 5, 179-182.

Walraven, J.(1982). Tast- en steunstokken voor visueel gehandicapten; een inventarisatie en evaluatie van functionele, ergonomische en mechanische aspecten. IZF report 1982-C15, Institute for Perception, Soesterberg, The Netherlands.

Wilson, J.P. (1966). Obstacle detection using ambient or self-generated noise. Nature 211, 218.

THE ROLE OF EVALUATION AND OF INSPIRATION IN THE DEVELOPMENT OF
ELECTRONIC TRAVEL AIDS FOR THE BLIND

A.D. Heyes
Blind Mobility Research Unit
University of Nottingham, England

Introduction.

My aim in this paper is to present what I consider to be
the essential ingredients for success in the development of
electronic travel aids for the blind. I will illustrate
several points by reference to the Sonic Pathfinder, (Heyes,
1984) an aid recently developed in Nottingham. Because this
is a 'Workshop' and not a conference I feel it inappropiate to
present a formal paper. Instead I will take the opportunity
to put a personal view as to how best to conduct research in
this important area. If it is the feeling of the meeting that
my views do point the way forward, then I will have made a
useful contribution. If, however, this is not the feeling, at
least I should have stimulated a valuable discussion.

The two philosophies.

It is possible to identify two distinct philosophical
attitudes to the problem of aid development.

The traditional attitude, I call it the engineers'
attitude, may be articulated as follows:- the reason why the
blind have difficulty in getting around is because they lack
the visual information that is necessary. Clearly what is
required is to collect this information, process it, and feed
it to one of the remaining senses or even directly to the
visual cortex. Reference is made to psychology, in particular
to the fact that the human central nervous system has been
found to be remarkably good at processing distorted
information and in selectively attending to what is relevent.
A consequence of this is reluctance to discard information in
the belief that, even if the display is complicated, the blind
will, in time, learn to find it useful. An early example of
the application of this design philosophy was the Sonic Torch
(Kay, 1964). So much has been written about this device,
suffice it to recall that the aid uses ultra-sonics and
produces an information rich sound display which relates to
the range and the surface texture of all the objects within
the area viewed by the beam. This is impressive. One can

point the aid at successive objects: a tree, a wall, a car, etc. and imagine the blind user being able to learn a vocabulary of sound signatures corresponding to these objects. Unfortunately, the results with the blind were a bitter disappointment; very few were able to obtain enough information from the aid to ensure its continued use. In commercial terms the aid was a failure; of the 1,000 devices made less than 100 were sold. As a direct result of this, British manufacturers have since shown considerable reluctance to become involved with mobility aids for the blind. The dilemma of an aid which offered so much potential and yet proved so difficult to use attracted the attention of many psychologists. The main result being the production of a large training manual.

One psychologist attracted to the problem was the late J. Alfred Leonard. His analysis has led to a radically different philosophical approach to aid development. His starting point was the simple, but very relevent, observation that there were some blind people who could get on very well without the use of clever electronic devices. He argued that not until we could understand blind mobility could we hope to improve it. He became an enthusiastic supporter of the long cane and played an important role in its introduction to the United Kingdom. He gathered around him a small group of psychologists, insisted that they all underwent long cane training under the blindfold and set about the task of devising mobility evaluation techniques capable of giving an objective measure of the performance of the blind man and his aid. He established the Blind Mobility Research Unit at Nottingham, where his original ideas on evaluation have been translated into a very effective technique of aid assesment, (Dodds, Carter & Howarth, 1983).

My arrival, as a physicist, at Nottingham led to a period of aid development along lines anticipated by Leonard. No attempt was made to devise a surrogate for vision, rather a series of simple devices were produced which were designed to give the user limited additional information to that provided by his remaining senses. Each developmental step was followed by a period of evaluation using blind volunteers; the experience gained during the evaluation being used to give an insight as to the next design step. This procedure of alternate periods of aid development and evaluation forms the basis of the alternative design philosophy. Progress is slow but measurable and finite.

The two different design philosophies have led to aids being categorised as either environment sensors or obstacle detectors.

Aids continue to be designed using both philosophical approaches. The engineers continue to make unwarrented assumptions about the information processing capabilities of the blind pedestrian, but, do the psychologists do any better? My latest aid, the Sonic Pathfinder, is a direct product of the interactive research programme carried out in Nottingham. It appears, on the basis of our evaluation, to provide most of the relevent information necessary for safe and efficient travel. It represents a major step forward from our previous hand held device, but this step has not been taken as smoothly as was anticipated by Leonard. There is a major flaw in his assumption that the results of an evaluation would feed DIRECTLY into the next development. He failed to describe the mechanism and role of inspiration.

The mechanism of inspiration.

Crossing the bridge between the findings of one evaluation and the design of the next device involves an element of inspiration. I believe that the technique that I have evolved for obtaining this inspiration can be used by others. Therefore I propose to disclose my somewhat idiosyncratic technique.

The Nottingham evaluation procedure involves video-taping the blind subjects walking over a typical outdoor route both with and without the aid. The analysis of these tapes, carried out by my colleagues, involves scoring the performance under a number of headings. For instance, counting the number of cane and body contacts with objects and estimating the amount of time spent travelling in the required direction compared to that spent reorientating. The resulting profile gives a good measure of the value of the aid. I have no complaint either with the procedure or with the results obtained. However, although this procedure will highlight any defects in the aid it does not tell me, the designer, how to implement inprovements. My idiosyncratic technique of solving this problem involves spending just as much time looking at the tapes but paying particular attention to the difficulties encountered by the users. I then drive out to the route, get myself into the difficult situations, and ask myself just what is the information I need to resolve the difficulty.

The example.

The Sonic Pathfinder is a spectacle-frame-mounted ultra-sonic pulse-echo device with an auditory display. The prime function is to detect and indicate the

distance of any obstacle which lies directly in the
blind pedestrian's path. In the absence of any
obstruction ahead, it reverts to its secondary function
of indicating the presence and range of obstacles to the
left and right of the travel path. The aid represents
the distance of the nearest object in terms of the notes
of the musical scale - one note being assigned to each
of the 300 mm. (1ft.) range zones. It is a digital
device; no attempt being made to provide an analogue
signal giving textural information. This is done to
avoid information overload. The user listens to the
display through two small earpieces, one mounted on each
side of the spectacle frame in close proximity to,
though not actually in contact with, the ear. Time
division multiplexing is employed between the three
receivers and the two earpieces so that the distance of
any object which lies, within range, to the left of the
main travel path is signalled only in the left earpiece
whilst an object to the right is signalled only in the
right earpiece. An object which lies directly ahead
produces a signal at both earpieces thus creating a
central sound image. In the absence of any obstacle
within the area viewed by the aid the display is totally
silent.

When in use the pedestrian is able to walk parallel to
the inner shore line - a hedge or wall - by keeping the
repeating note at the 'inner' ear at a constant pitch.
He is at the same time able to tell when he passes a
tree or lamp-post on the outer shore-line by the
interposition of the occasional note in the other ear;
such objects are vital landmarks for the blind. If he
encounters an object lying directly ahead, the side
information is no longer provided - Centre Echo Priority
- and information relating to the central hazard is
presented to both ears. As an additional 'attention
grabber' the central display is arranged to have a
repetition rate four times that for the side information
- 16 times a second. Only when the hazard is
circumnavigated does the aid revert to giving side
information.

A number of prototypes have been evaluated using blind
volunteers, (Dodds, Carter and Howarth, in press). The
results encourage me in the belief that we are following
the correct philosophical approach. Some shortcomings
were identified during the evaluation. For example, it
was known before hand that the aid was difficult to use
in cluttered environments. A range switch had been
fitted and users advised to switch from long to short

range - ie. from 2.4 metres (8ft.) down to 1.2 metres (4ft.) - when trying to negotiate narrow openings. The evaluation showed that subjects ignored this advice! Additional training might produce more optimal use, however, by changing to a microprocessor based system and using the techniques discribed in this paper I have been able to develop software information processing algorithms which achieve an automatic adjustment of the range.

The difficulties encountered during the evaluation by users trying to negotiate narrow gaps may be illustrated with reference to Figure 1. The figure depicts a plan view of a subject standing still and facing an open doorway leading onto a corridor. Very small rotations of the head produce three different musical notes: a note of low pitch corresponding to the distance to the nearest door-post $d1$, a note of higher pitch corresponding to the distance to the corridor wall w, and a note of intermediate pitch corresponding to the distance to the far door-post $d2$. The Centre Echo Priority algorithm ensures that these notes are presented to both ears giving no obvious impression of the existence of a gap. Furthermore, very small head movements produce a jangling sound which is very difficult to interpret. (The user will only realise he is facing a gap when he notices that one of the notes has a higher pitch than the other two!) How much better the information display would be if the aid had a maximum range greater than $d2$ but less than w! If this were the case small head rotations would produce: a note of low pitch corresponding to distance $d1$, a note of higher pitch corresponding to distance $d2$, and a middle position in which these two notes are presented alternately to the left and right ears giving an unambiguous indication of an opening in the centre.

I have achieved this display by the introduction of an algorithm which I have named the Ratchet. Essentially the action of the Ratchet is to reduce the range of the aid to that of the nearest object in the central region and to maintain this limited range for a certain time, the Ratchet Hold Time. In order to avoid numerous undesirable side-effects certain constraints must be placed on the Ratchet algorithm. For instance, refering to Figure 1, a crude Ratchet with a hold time greater than, say, 2 seconds would result in the near door-post - the note corresponding to the distance $d1$ - alone being displayed. This seems inappropriate since the far door-post - distance $d2$ - is sufficiently close that it could be encountered within the 2 second hold time, even if, as in this case, the subject is moving from a standing start. Consideration of walking speed, acceleration and reaction times have led to the action of the Ratchet being restricted to the four outer zones of the aid. Thus the Ratchet never reduces the range of the aid to less than 1.2 metres (4ft.).

A careful choice of Ratchet Hold Time is crucial if other undesirable side-effects are to be avoided. In the above example a Ratchet Hold Time of 2 seconds was chosen. A duration which is long compared to the time taken for the user to make head rotations but short compared to the time required to negotiate the doorway and move into the comparative open space of the corridor. Although in these circumstances the choice of 2 seconds for the Ratchet Hold Time is appropriate it does, however, produce one unfortunate consequence. If a user is using the side signal of the aid in order to maintain a travel line parallel to the shore line at a distance of say 90 mm. (3ft.), and if he were momentarily to rotate his head towards the shore line, the Ratchet would immediately be invoked and the range of the aid set to 1.2 metres (4ft.). (1.2 meters (4ft) not 90 mm. (3ft), because of the restriction described above.) Thus from that moment, for the duration of the Ratchet Hold Time, the user has only the protection of an aid with a range of 1.2 metres (4ft). In these circumstances this is serious because he is not moving from a standing start, he may be travelling at 6 km/h. (4mph)! The solution is to use a Ratchet Hold Time proportional to the time the invoking object remained in 'view'. Thus a quick 'glance' towards a near object would produce a hold time considerably shorter than would a prolonged 'stare'. It does, however, remain necessary to limit the Ratchet Hold Time to some maximum value - 2 seconds seems to be appropriate.

Having made the Ratchet Hold Time dynamically determined one has, in effect, produced an aid, the range of which is governed by the walking speed of the user. That is to say, instead of an aid with a range of 2.4 metres (8ft), we have an aid with a range of 2 seconds! Rather an odd concept. However, given the information processing demands inherent in independent blind travel (Shingledecker, 1978) and the moment to moment problem solving nature of blind travel (Dodds, personal communication) it would seem highly desirable to have an aid which was limited to providing information solely about those objects which would be encountered during the next 2 seconds of travel.

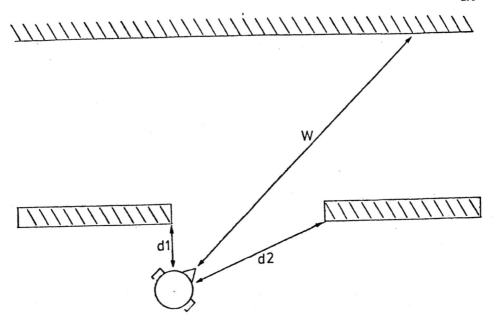

FIGURE 1 PLAN VIEW OF USER APPROACHING AN OPEN DOORWAY

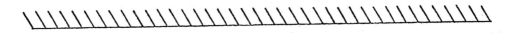

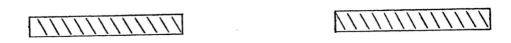

FIGURE 2 USER ABOUT TO PASS THROUGH OPEN DOORWAY

Figure 2 illustrates what may happen when our blind subject takes a pace forward. Large head rotations are now required to bring the door-posts into the central region of the aid and there is a high probability that the Ratchet will be released before the doorway is negotiated. When this happens the aid returns to having a 2.4 metres (8ft) range and the Centre Echo Priority algorithm ensures that the musical note corresponding to the corridor wall is displayed, rather than the side information about the door-posts. The undesirable effect may be eliminated by yet another information processing algorithm - the Clamp.

The Ratchet is only be invoked and sustained by signals received in the central, forward facing receiver. The Clamp, on the other hand, may be invoked and sustained by any signal received in the nearest zone of the aid (zone 1) whether left, right or centre. The Clamp operates for a fixed duration (1.2 seconds) and has the effect of reducing the aid to a single zone device. By increasing the length of near zone to just less than arms' length and reducing the ranges of the other zones so that the overall range of the aid remains equal to 2.4 metres (8ft) the Clamp provides an effective solution to the problem described with reference to Figure 2. The presence of one or the other door-post in the side regions of the near zone prevents the far corridor wall from being perceived no matter how slowly the subject moves. Only when he steps through the doorway is the user informed of the existence of the corridor wall. Indeed, it is only then that this information becomes relevant.

After introducing the Clamp it became necessary to reduce the maximum Ratchet Hold Time to 1.5 seconds. This is because the Clamp and the Ratchet are additive.

The existence of the Ratchet and the Clamp will not be perceived by the user during normal use of the Sonic Pathfinder. The various durations used in the algorithms have been chosen to correspond to those involved in human movement. Consequently, the user does not, contrary to what might appear to be the case from the above description, experience objects leaping in and out of his perception. There is only one weird side-effect; all objects disappear if the user walks backwards!

I propose the Ratchet and the Clamp as a solution to the problems highlighted by the evaluation. We now need another evaluation to discover whether my conjecture is correct! The point I wish to make is that the simple procedure of using the aid allowed me to generate a number of testable hyphotheses thus enabling the research programme to move forward. This seems to be an obvious way to proceed and yet it has attracted considerable criticism. Why is this? I fully accept that a few minutes using the aid does not enable one to make a judgement as to the aid's value; our evaluation procedure does this. The answer is that psychologists are suspicious of introspection. This is not without good reason; the history of the subject is littered with mistaken insij...s obtained in this way. What I would like is for psychologists to reinstate introspection; take the inherent risks and use it to generate testable conjectures. I would maintain that mistakes don't matter, the subsequent evaluation will allow the utility or otherwise of any modification to be assessed. The irony is that engineers frequently use introspection and yet because they lack the psychologists' knowledge of perceptual theory they are not the best people to make use of it.

Conclusions.

My recipe for progress is simple. Both engineers and psycholgists have much to offer but the engineers must be prepared to subject their ideas to the sort of objective evaluations developed by psychologists. Meanwhile the psychologists must, if they wish to make a contribution at the design stage, be prepared to overcome their prejudice against introspection.

Acknowledgments.

The Blind Mobility Research Unit is sustained by the Department of Health and Social Service and is directed by Professor C. I. Howarth. I am grateful for the support they have given to my work.

296

References.

Dodds A.G., Carter C.C. & Howarth C.I. (1983) 'Improving Objective Measures of Mobility'. Journal of Visual Impairment and Blindness, Vol.77, No.9 pp.438-442.

Heyes A.D. (1984) 'The Sonic Pathfinder'. Electronics and Wireless World, Vol.90, No.1579, pp.26-29 & 62.

Kay L. (1964) 'An Ultra-sonic probe as a mobility aid for the blind'. Ultrasonics, April-June, pp.53-59.

Shingledecker C.A. (1978) 'The effects of anticipation on performance and processing load on blind mobility'. Ergonomics Vol.21, pp.335-371.

DEVELOPMENT AND EVALUATION OF MOBILITY AIDS FOR THE VISUALLY HANDICAPPED

G. Jansson
Department of Psychology
University of Uppsala, Sweden

CONTENTS

ENGINEERING AND KNOWLEDGE ABOUT PERCEPTION

A perceptual aid and its user form a system which aims to make it possible for the user to pick up information from the environment. In order to successfully perform this task, the necessary information must, of course, be available via the aid, but that is not sufficient. The information must also have a useful form. Often it is difficult for the user to pick up the artificial information at first when trying to use the aid. The constructor has to rely upon the great adaptability of the human being, and in many cases she can learn to pick up the new information successfully after adequate training.

However, in many cases electronic mobility aids intended to supplement primary aids such as a long cane or a guide dog do not seem to work satisfactorily. This is indicated by the rather low number of users in spite of the many years such aids have been available (Table 1) as well as by the high proportion of drop-outs from training and use of the aid (Table 2).

There are many factors affecting figures of this kind, but the following two hypothesis point to some probably significant contributing factors: (a) the information made available does not contain a satisfying amount of the information needed, and (b) the form of this information is not sufficiently adapted to the functioning of the perceptual system involved. It is very probable that the availability of more adequate information and/or a form of the available information more adapted to the human system involved should increase the number of people beginning to use the aid as well as decrease the proportion of drop-outs.

For the development of mobility aids for the visually handicapped the constructor should have knowledge of at least the following problem areas : (1) the information needed by a pedestrian for successful travelling, (2) the technically possible ways of displaying that information in a non-visual form, and (3) the usefulness of these alternative displays for a human user.

The most readily accessible knowledge is the technical one. Knowledge about the perceptual aspects is more difficult to attain because it often requires time-consuming theoretical and experimental work, especially if a more general coverage of the problem area is wanted. The development of aids can hardly wait for a "complete" solution, but it is important that the knowledge available now about perceptual factors is maximally utilized in the construction process.

So far, this knowledge has not been extensively utilized. Typically, mobility aids have been developed by concerned mobility teachers or people with engineering insights. Perceptual points of view have probably been considered in most aid-construction contexts, at least to some extent, but technical aspects have dominated. When stating this I will not pretend that we should have had perfect aids if more perceptual knowledge had been introduced, but I think that some not very successful technical alternatives would have been dropped earlier, and some more promising alternatives would have been tried. A closer cooperation between engineering and perception experts is an interesting option for the future. To give rules for such a cooperative effort is impossible, as the form depends to such a degree on many different circumstances. Let me here only make a few general remarks.

Table 1. Number of students who had so far completed their training within the Veterans Administration, USA, on each of the mobility aids (Leicester W. Farmer, personal communication, 1980).

Sonic Guide	70
American Laser Cane	32
Pathsounder	8
Mowat Sensor	15
Total	125

Table 2. Number of students within the Veterans Administration, USA, being trained on the American Laser Cane and using the aid after training (Leicester W. Farmer, personal communication, 1980).

Starting training	37
Completing training	32
Keeping the aid immediately after training	22
Still using the aid one year after training	17

PERCEPTION RESEARCH DURING THE CONSTRUCTION PHASE

During the construction phase, perceptual theory may contribute to the discussion of what kinds of information might be useful for a new device. At this point the possibilities of the existing aids, as well as information wanted to be available in an ideal aid, should be compared with what information the new aid can give. Can the new aid be expected to make a significant addition, or be a successful substitute for some of the available aids? It seems that it is common with a too-optimistic judgment concerning the possibilities of a new aid. An analysis of what information it makes available and of how useful the planned display of this information can be expected to be may save much effort and decrease the risk of developing aids with little prospect of success.

Another kind of contribution of knowledge about perception concerns the choice between alternative displays. In some cases there might be easily obtainable knowledge about the suitability of the alternatives considered, but usually experiments have to be performed. This is especially apparent when non-natural kinds of stimulation, such as electrocutaneous stimulation, are contemplated (cf. Szeto & Saunders, 1982). The delays in the engineering work that studies of this kind may lead to can probably explain why they are not more common. The constructor may prefer to guess or to make some very informal experiment instead of waiting for a carefully performed study. It may work sometimes, but it may also lead to futile work along unsuccessful lines.

The experimental study to be made does not need to be concerned with the whole task of walking, but with smaller or larger aspects of this task. Therefore, the experiment in this context must not necessarily be performed with a final aid, but with simpler equipment displaying only the information of immediate interest. It may also be possible to present the perceptual alternatives by computer simulation (cf. Tachi, Mann & Rowell, 1983). In other cases it may be necessary to build a relatively advanced prototype, e.g. when the display is a large matrix of tactile point stimuli. Typically the study is an experiment performed indoors in a well-controlled environment.

EVALUATION OF EXISTING AIDS

It is easier to indicate the forms of evaluations of already existing aids (or prototypes) than the forms of perception research during the construction phase. This is a more traditional type of applied psychology, and several different methods have been developed. They will be discussed in three groups: (1) free use, (2) field experiments, and (3) laboratory experiments. (For a differently structured but in many respects related discussion, see Shingledecker and Foulke, 1978).

Free use.

This is probably the most common method, but also the least reliable one. By free use I mean a study in which a user is given an aid for use in his daily life with a general instruction to evaluate it. He may or may not be given an instruction in how to use it. The result depends very much on his capacity for self-instruction. Other random factors both within the evaluator and in his environment may have great effects, such as his motivation and walking habits, as well as special features of the evaluator's environment and non-representative events happening during the evaluation period. This method can be made more reliable by the use of many evaluators, by adequate training in the use of the aid, and by a careful procedure for the collection of data (e.g. by daily reports and/or well-planned interviews), but with this method it is not possible to avoid a great influence of random factors.

The main advantage of the free-use method, and probably the main reason for its popularity, is that the aid is used in a natural environment. Thus, the aid has to demonstrate its usefulness in the full complexity of natural life. Therefore, this method, in spite of all its weaknesses, might be suitable for a final evaluation of an aid just before its release for more general use. Earlier studies of the aid may have been concerned only with restricted aspects of human performance with the aid. In a free-use study the complex interaction of all relevant factors is given a chance to affect the performance. This type of evaluation may also demonstrate important aspects that have not been considered during the earlier work with the device. Therefore a free-use study may have an important function to fulfil at a late stage in the development of an aid, but its weaknesses must be remembered, and it should never be the only method used.

Field experiments

One way of decreasing the effects of random factors is to study the use of the aid in specially chosen environments; in the case of field experiments, this means natural environments. Such a method for mobility aids for the visually handicapped has been developed at Blind Mobility Research Unit, Nottingham University, England (Armstrong, 1975). After a period of training in how to use the aid, the user walks a special route which has been chosen as reasonably representative of many environments encountered by blind pedestrians. He walks the route both with and without the aid studied, and his locomotion is videotaped. These recordings are analysed in several parameters indicating with what safety, efficiency, and stress the traveller performs his task.

By this method it is possible to get a nuanced judgment in what respects the aid has been helpful. Because of the greater control of the situation compared with the free-use method, this method is less affected by random factors, but as the study is made in a real-world setting there is a possibility of unintended events and situations affecting the result, such as playing children and cars parked on the sidewalk. The great advantage of this method is in the possibility of measuring the behavior of the pedestrian in an objective way.

Laboratory experiments

The significant feature of this type of investigation is that it involves a higher degree of control of the whole situation studied. Therefore, more reliable results can be obtained, but, as in all laboratory studies, there is a risk of not being able to generalize the results to the more complex real situations.

The laboratory experiments may have an enormous variety of forms, but preferably they should be planned within the framework of a general theory of the perceptual guidance of locomotion. Unfortunately, there is no such well-established theory, but outlines to a theory in this area are available, and these should be maximally utilized in the analysing of the problems and the planning of the experiments. I prefer to elaborate on the outline given by Gibson (1979), and I have elsewhere (Jansson, in press) discussed this in some detail.

I think that the following aspects of walking are among the most important ones: (1) keeping balance, (2) walking towards a goal, (3) walking along a guideline, and (4) walking around obstacles. To work within the framework of such an outline means that the experimental situations considered are analysed in terms of these basic aspects. E.g., in the evaluation of the Swedish Laser Cane (Jansson, 1975) I studied a subaspect of walking around an obstacle, i.e. the detection of the obstacle. In evaluations of the Electrophthalm and the Tactile Vision Substitution System (Jansson, 1983) the aspect studied was walking towards a goal, and in a recent evaluation of an electronic guideline digged into the ground (Jansson, unpublished experiment) it was walking along a guideline.

The general theoretical framework has less to contribute to experiments on the _form_ of the information. In that context more specific theories of the sense considered may be more helpful. But often the theoretical contexts do not include such important aspects as dynamic stimulation and the function of the information for the guidance of movement, and so there may be necessary to make new experiments encompassing these aspects.

It should be noted that laboratory experiments on this kind of problem may contain much real walking, and therefore often need larger spaces than usually used in behavioral studies. Treadmills are often not appropriate as they do not allow the subject to have control over the direction of his walking.

In addition to the increased control over experimental conditions, the laboratory method gives you a possibility to search for specific information limitations of a device or a prototype in a meaningful way. An analysis of the devices developed so far (cf. Jansson, in press) indicates that a major deficiency is that no aid can guide a pedestrian toward a goal at longer distances than a few meters. The blind person has to rely, to a very large extent, on walking along some guideline, either existing without special regard to the blind person's needs (such as a hedge, a curb, or an edge between two different kinds of ground material) or specially built to be helpful for blind mobility (such as certain electronic guidelines).

One problem that has been observed in connection with

several evaluations is that differences between the performances with and without an aid may not show up in objective measures (cf. Dodds, Carter & Howarth, 1983). One interpretation of such results is that the measures are not sensitive enough to discriminate between the conditions. Another possible interpretation is, of course, that there are no important differences in these cases. I personally tend to favor the latter hypothesis. The electronic aids developed so far are not very effective, and it might very well be that adding them to the primary aid has no great effect. To be practically interesting, an aid should add substantially to the performance possible without the aid. It is therefore more important to find perceptual conditions giving such a very evident effect than to make the methods more sensitive.

Choice of method

    The three groups of methods discussed above can to a large extent be seen as complements to each other. The free-use method, especially if a more sophisticated version is used, is suitable when the usefulness of a final aid is tried just before its introduction to a larger population. The laboratory experiment method, with its possibilities of giving answers to very specific questions, is the most useful method when looking for a detailed understanding of the function of a (potential) aid. It should be the main method during the construction phase (cf. above), and it has probably its greatest importance during the early phases of the development of an aid. The field experiment may be used for a final aid or an early prototype. It can be seen as an alternative to the free-use method when more objective measurements are wanted.

Concluding remarks
==================

    The psychology of perception has thus far contributed to the scientific work on mobility aids for the visually handicapped mainly by taking part in the evaluation of final aids or late prototypes. This is an important task which can be made still better if the methods are refined, especially if the evaluation is made in a theoretical context. However, a still more important task is to take part in the development of new aids by contributing earlier to the work on the aid. The psychology of perception can add to the discussions on what information should be made available with the aid and on what forms of this information can be expected to be most efficient.

ACKNOWLEDGEMENTS
================

    My work in this area was made possible by grants from the Bank of Sweden Tercentenary Foundation (dnr 75/116, 81/96), from the Swedish Council for the Humanities and the Social Sciences (dnr F 926/78, 615/79, 452/80, 417/82), and from the Delegation for Social Research (dnr 82/117).

REFERENCES

Armstrong, J. D. (1975). Evaluation of man-machine systems in the mobility of the visually handicapped. In R. M. Pickett & T. J. Triggs (Eds.), Human factors in health care (pp. 331-343). Lexington, MA: Heath.

Dodds, A. G., Carter, D. D. C., & Howarth, C. J. (1983). Improving objective measures of mobility. Journal of Visual Impairment and Blindness, 77, 438-442.

Gibson, J. J. (1979). The ecological approach to visual perception. Boston, MA: Houghton Mifflin.

Jansson, G. (1975). The detection of objects by the blind with the aid of a laser cane (Report No. 172). Uppsala, Sweden: University of Uppsala, Department of Psychology.

Jansson, G. (1983) Tactile guidance of movement. International Journal of Neuroscience, 19, 37-46.

Jansson, G. (In press). Perceptual theory and sensory substitution. In D. Ingle, M. Jeannerod, & D. Lee (Eds.), Brain mechanisms and spatial vision. The Hague, the Netherlands: Nijhoff.

Shingledecker, C. A. & Foulke, E. (1978). A human factors approach to the assessment of the mobility of blind pedestrians. Human factors, 20, 273-286.

Szeto, A. Y. T. & Saunders, F. A. (1982). Electrocutaneous stimulation for sensory communication in rehabilitation engineering. IEEE Transactions on Biomedical Engineering, BME-29, 300-308.

Tachi, S., Mann, R. W., & Rowell, D. (1983). Quantitative comparison of alternative sensory displays for mobility aids for the blind. IEEE Transactions on Biomedical Engineering, BME-30 571-577.

DISCUSSION

Orban

I would like to make a couple of comments. First of all, I think, we have here a nice example of how physiology can help. I think that the "echolocating" device like the one Dr. Heyes presented, the sonic aid, was inspired from physiology but a physiology which is not ours but that of the bat. The bat has a beautiful system that works along those lines: it sends out ultrasounds and it takes in the signals, and has special sensory centers to process them. Some of the problems arise from trying to apply that kind of processing to our auditory channel which is made in a different way. The second comment I want to make is that here we are talking about mobility rather than object recognition. This an important distinction, I think, space localization of an object and object recognition. The auditory system may be not the most suited to provide spatial localization. At the level of the receptor, at the cochlea, all explicit information on spatial localization is lost. We have in our auditory system - further in the brain - special centers to recreate that information, but this is achieved only partially, and it is achieved by comparing the signals from the two ears. So, we will always need the two ears - I think you made some comments on the "binaurality". So, that's how our auditory system works. Also, the result of that computation is, as I said, imperfect. It is ambiguous. The way to solve this is by moving our head. So, I am not sure that, if we are really interested in mobility, the choice of auditory substitution is optimal.

Werner (to Bruun)

May I rise a general question to the physiologist? Is there any research and are there results which could tell us how much logic you have to put into these channels? We are trying to substitute the channels of communication provided by the eyes. The eyes apparently have a very broad band to communicate data, but that of the ear, I think, is comparatively narrow, it seems more or less one-dimensional. You have just the frequencies. The skin can accept intensities, perhaps. But it is again a one-dimensional scale. The question arises: is there any investigation on what interfaces could be used and how much they can be loaded with information, because the ear is also used for other purposes? E.g., if you are in the traffic, you have to take notice of alarms given by cars, etc.

Bruun

Well, I'm not the one to answer this question.

Heyes

One of the many things we've done in this area at Nottingham is
to look at the information processing capability of the blind
traveler. It's not just a question of measuring the different
types of input, whether with the ear or the skin. It is to do it
within the context of a man walking along the street. We have
measured channel capacity, and come to the conclusion that many
of the existing aids already overload channel capacity. Success
with mobility aids is going to largely depend upon choosing displays which are extremely simple to understand, very natural
displays, whether they be through the skin or whether they be
through the ear. We have arguments both for the skin and for the
ear. But, certainly, one has to be extraordinarily careful not
to overload the sensory channel capacity of the blind. Being
independent and mobile and blind is extraordinarily stressful.
Blind people do not walk along the street day-dreaming, they
walk along the street working very hard. They are constantly
generating hypotheses about the next step. This is a very stressful business, and we are measuring that stress.

Bruun

Even if I am not a psychologist, I would like once more to stress
the importance of the learning curve - when evaluating new aids.
Remember how long time it takes a small child to learn to see
and hear. For many new aids the users will probably never get to
the flat part of the learning curve.

Levett

I think it's interesting as we switch back and forth from physical systems to neurophysiological systems. It's interesting, I
think, to build in some of the analogies. For example, we switch
from auditory to visual. If we change in orientation, the visual
system is capable of recognizing the same object. The auditory
system, if we "switch" in pitch, recognizes the same melody.
Perhaps, in considering some of these kinds of things, it will
help us with the development of our technology. Also to recognize
some of the things that are happening in other areas. It struck
me when Dr. Orban was talking about a number of things. There is
now a new ejection seat, in offence technology. Some microwave
computations that are built in enable its orientation to be
specified. This is of vital importance, if the pilot ejects when
the plane is upside down. A measure of the microwave intensity
from the sky as opposed to the ground produces a difference signal and therefore we can make a "binaural" estimation or, if
you will, a comparison for orientation specification. Dr. Powell's
talk this morning led back to some of the early work that went on
in the frog, in the visual edge detectors, that came out of MIT,

and to the interesting observation that only when it passed
through the edge you got a frequency blip. In the neural system
we are only interested in rates of changes essentially. When
things are constant we don't want a lot of processing to be
going on, because that would be uneconomical. Only when we have
a change, that is an edge is imposed in the path, then, of
course, the frequency changes or in the presentation the second
note was heard. At least that's how I detected it, and it re-
minded me of the edge detector. I wonder what happens in your
system (instead of having that kind of manipulation), if now you
move the edge in space and look at the transfer function, when
you change object and target.

Bruun (to Walraven)

The long white cane is the most important mobility aid. Even when
we provide a blind user with the best elctronic aid he will not
like to be without the cane, - I am sure he will prefer the cane
to any device we've seen up to now. This holds in particular for
those who were born blind.

Heyes

If you compare an electronic mobility aid to a long cane, it is
significant to realize that the difference in independent mobility achieved by the blind person before and after he receives
long cane training, is really very large indeed. Whereas the
difference that he gets from the extra addition of a high technology aid, on top of his long cane, is really not all that great.
I wish it were otherwise, but I think it's true, the long cane
is going to be here for a very, very long time to come, and it's
a super mobility aid.

Jansson

May be I should just add that we've made some experiments on the
performance with a cane of this kind. We made physical measurements of the sounds of a series of canes, and we found a lot of
differences in the acoustical parameters. Then we studied the
same canes in a behavioural situation where the subjects should
detect and localize objects, and in this situation we didn't
find, to our surprise, any differences between the canes. My interpretation of this fact is that, even if there are a lot of
acoustical differences, they may not be important in the practical situation, e.g. the differences may be masked by all the
reverberations you have in an ordinary room. There are a lot of
experiments still to be done, but it's clear that the "hope" you
may get from physical measurements alone may not show up in behavioural experiments.

Thomsen

When you told about further development in electronics, trav-

elling with mobility aids, I think for scientists and researchers
it's very important to keep in mind that, with the long cane, the
blind user has got a cheap and simple travelling aid. Prof. Bruun
asked for a "curve" detector. Well, if you know how to use the
long cane, you have an excellent tool for curve detection. To my
opinion, the only inconvenience with the long cane is, when you
have to find a place for dinner, a restaurant. But the greatest
inconvenience is that it takes so long time to learn to use a
long cane. You have to go through a program for 3 to 6 months before you can achieve this goal. Anyway, you can use the long cane
safely in the environment, whether you are a young, physically
fit person or you are an old person, say, 80 years old. You can
use the same tool for moving around independently and safely.

Orban (to Jansson)

I certainly think that there is no antinomy between our approaches.
You too stressed the importance of the conceptualization before
the design or during the design, and I think the brain is such a
very complex organ that physiology is not enough. We need several
means of approaching it. I think the perceptual aspects are extremely valuable. It is just pointing exactly to the same direction. The last transparency is a further illustration of what I
said, that is we should enable the blind to manipulate his visual
environment. This is much more than just avoiding obstacles.

Jansson

I very much agree to that. I see the physiological and the perceptual approaches as complementary. We have different theoretical contexts to take our knowledge from.

Tobin

I'm a bit fearful that we should be holding this kind of workshop
in ten years time, twenty years time; that is, the physiologists
and psychologists, the engineers, the rehabilitation experts and
educators will come together again, and the Dr. Orbans, and Dr.
Janssons, and people like myself would be coming along and saying: you haven't taken account, you engineers, of this. You,
engineers, would be saying: you haven't got involved with us.
I'm really fearful that there will just be an endless series of
this kind of discussion, and then we will each go away into our
own little boxes. I think we must do something about that, Dr.
Emiliani, before the end of the day, at least in the sense of
making recommendations. I think most of you have identified me
with Dr. Orban and Dr. Jansson, at least in the sense that we
were arguing that more knowledge is needed about the human organism, so that that knowledge can be built into the system.
But that really is doing an injustice, I think, to us three and
to the rest of you. It isn't as simple as that. It seems to me
that we cannot assume that the right approach is to develop

knowledge about how the human organism works, and then to build
that into some engineering device, because it would put all you
engineers out of work for many years to come until we have
solved these problems. We know that in fact progress is made in
the absence of complete knowledge. I mean, if you want to look
at the brain of the human neonate and then separately look at
human languages, natural languages, we would all say: it is impossible for a five years old child to be able to speak. Human
languages are much too complex for a five years old to be able
to communicate in French or German or English or Swedish. We
would say that we need to know a lot more about languages and a
lot more about the human brain and the human organism before we
can get the five years old to speak. And yet even educationally
subnormal children, who find difficult to add 7 to 8, communicate very effectively, don't they? They speak and they exchange
information with people of their own age and older. In other
words, in the absence of complete knowledge about the structure
of human languages and how the human brain processes the information, things happen. What am I arguing is that, we must let
the engineers push ahead, otherwise we should lose their energy
and their ideas, and we must keep on saying that the psychologists and physiologists must be doing their work, so that
their work can inform the product. I want to suggest that both
come together; in fact, it isn't the case of which comes first.
The chicken and the egg exist together, at the moment. It's not
useful to argue who should come first and which does come first.
It's a sheer fact, the two things have got to go on together.
I think the question is: how do we insure that the kind of information that is getting exchanged in meetings like this, then
gets implemented in the next generation of devices? It seems
to me we are not addressing that problem at all, because each
of us will go back to our own countries, will be heavily dependent upon our present levels of funding and we will be getting
on with our own work, and we will pay lip-service to the need
for this interdisciplinary approach. And I suspect we'll do no
more than pay lip-service. We will it have the back of our minds,
and we shan't have it within the structures in which we are actually working, I suggest.

Orban

Of course, I agree, with Dr. Tobin, he is perfectly right. We
have short- and long-term strategies. The only thing that I, and
probably Dr. Jansson, would like to avoid is that people would
go away and say: OK, it is all very well what these physiologists
and these psychologists do, but it will come too late, and so we
don't have to do anything about the long-term. I fully agree
that there is a short-term need for immediate action. We must of
course recognize this need, but in addition we must start the
long-term projects and emphasize that point and the need here.

If we push back the long-term projects, it will take even more
time, so the sooner we start and the more energy we put into them
the sooner we will get results.

Jansson

Just one addition which is on the same lines. I've found it very
fruitful to work on both ends of this dimension of applicability
and theoretical research. I've worked on these concrete aids rather much, but I've found it also very useful, originally coming
from a theoretical context, to work on the theoretical side of it.
So, I think it can very well be combined in one person to work
on concrete aids and on theoretical aspects. It might be fruitful;
you get ideas about theory when you work on concrete aids, and
the other way round.

Bruun

May I mention one problem which we have not included in the topics
at this workshop: the development of aids for orientation. Blind
persons need some aids to help them telling in which street they
are, where the corner is located, etc. I am not sure which technique should be used to communicate the information, it might be
ultrared light. In Sweden special sound signals are used to indicate street crossings and the state of light signals. In order
to get some acceptance of the costs of providing orientation aids
we could hope to find some system which would be of use also for
sighted people.

Levett

We all work within our own constraints, personal, funding, knowledge. This won't stop the engineers and psychologists from moving
forward. I would just like to underscore something that Prof.
Jansson said, in-keeping with what Dr. Orban says, about the correct conceptual framework. Once we have the correct conceptual
framework we have a better grip on the kinds of questions that we
can ask. An example was the Nobel Prize for Hodgin and Huxley in
which they define the actual nerve action potential experimentally and formulate a mathematical model based on flux flow and ex-
changes. Another group working in the United States had the correct mathematical formulation that is a fit, but it didn't lead
to the kinds of experimental questions that the Hodgin-Huxley
model led to. I think we are going through the same kind of situations or problems in health care systems. We are just beginning to get a better grip on what health care systems are and
therefore we are asking more important and perhaps more meaningful questions of the health care system. Perhaps the application
of new organizational theory will shed light on health care systems.

Thomsen

In this session, and in the previous session as well, we have
most of the time talked about how we can invent new devices or
new systems for the blind, so that he or she can compensate for
the lack of vision, or said in another way, adapt themselves in
a better and easier way to the environment, the sighted environment. I appreciated very much what Heyes said about this new
device, that we sighted people, whether we are scientists,reha-
bilitation officers, educators or what not, now know often too
little about how these new devices work in practice. I think it's
very important that we try these aids out, not so that we can
have a feeling of what it is to be blind, but we can have a feeling of how these aids work and what information they don't give
us. Now, there is another approach to this whole thing of invent-
ing new devices. Sometimes, I think we should concentrate our
efforts more in finding new devices to arrange our environment,
so that it would be easier for the blind to find these gaps you
were talking about and avoid only obstacles which are there, because we, as sighted people, have arranged our environment in a
way which is not very easy for blind people to get around, whether
we are talking about travelling or getting access, reading information or whatever it is. So, there is another approach for
technicians as well or engineers, to arrange the environment in a
more suitable way for the blind.

AUTHOR INDEX